100 DELICIOUS, BUDGET-FRIENDLY AND EASY TO MAKE RECIPES

D1045053

WHOLE FOOD

30-DAY DIET

COOKBOOK

30 days that will change your life

Step-by-Step Guide to Weight Loss, Reversing Disease, Improving Eating Habits, and Healthy Lifestyle

ISBN-13: 978-1976234521

ISBN-10: 1976234522

Table of Contents

Chapter 1: What is the Whole 30-day diet?

The Whole 30 diet is a monthly cleansing program created in 2009. It is assumed that following this diet can provide a "reset" of metabolism and change the person's attitude to food.

The program was developed based on the assumption that some product groups have a very negative impact on the health and physical endurance of a person. And, therefore, if you exclude these foods from the diet, you can significantly improve your health. Both physical and mental.

The main goal of many people following Whole 30 diet is losing weight. However, the program offers more than the usual weight loss. With its help, you can understand what products are specifically harmful to you.

For different people, the list of intolerable foods may be somewhat different. To me, the appeal of Whole 30 is that this experiment does not go beyond common sense if to compare with the other diets.

The first step to following a whole foods plant based diet is understanding what it means. To put it plain and straightforward, it involves filling a majority of your diet with foods that are not processed or refined and come directly from plants. They are foods that are as close as possible to their sources and are completely unmodified.

It is not a diet restricted solely to fruits and vegetables; there are many delicious alternatives to help you have a satisfying choice of foods to eat.

1. How the diet works

The idea behind the whole foods diet system is simple. The goal is to investigate how your body responds to certain foods, by first eliminating them and then slowly reinstating them after the 30 days are up.

Try and watch the reaction of your body. In this way, you can clearly identify which products are not useful for you. Milk may be behind your stomach trouble; honey may be the culprit when it comes to your runny nose.

The specifics can be a little tricky — for example, you can't eat peanuts, but you can eat almonds, also from all legumes, you can eat just green bean — but it's not as complicated as it seems.

By the way, you do not have to eat a 100% organic diet to follow the program; that is an entirely different topic. This is not to say that your entire foods cannot be organic; it is just not a prerequisite to qualify as full or natural.

Apparently, organic or locally grown food could provide you with the added benefit of eliminating harmful toxins and chemicals, which can further the health benefit of eating whole foods. So, be careful and read products labels.

To help you navigate your way through the clearance, here's a step-by-step guide to all the foods you can and can't eat during that 30 days.

2. List of allowed and prohibited products

What you cannot eat	What you can eat
Sugar and any of its substitutes, including "useful natural" one, for example, honey or stevia leaf. Instead of vanilla extract use vanilla bean powder	All varieties of meat, poultry, fish, and seafood
Cereals and everything that is made of cereals. Wheat, oats, rice, and also corn are forbidden in any form, including whole grains	Eggs
All legumes, except their green kinds like beans. Strictly prohibited soybean and all products in which it may be present	Fruits. Even dried fruits are allowed, although fresh ones are preferable
Dairy products, including fermented ones, such as yogurt or kefir. And also cheese	Any varieties of vegetables. Potatoes appeared on this list in 2013
Any flavoring additives, flavors, preservatives (except vinegar)	Nuts and seeds, except for peanuts
Harmful vegetable oils - corn, sunflower, soybean oils, etc. Not all mayonnaise is allowed, read the label or make your own	Healthy fats like butter, preferably, ghee. You can use duck fat as well as useful vegetable oils - olive, coconut
All industrially produced food, as there is at least one forbidden component in each of them	

3. The Whole Food shopping list

I remind you that all foods should be natural (organic is not a must, but the best option). Avoid factory-made products as they usually contain harmful substances such as MSG, sulfites, or added sugar.

Protein:

Minced beef/lamb/pork	Turkey
Beef/lamb/pork joint	Salmon
Sausages/bacon/ham*	Seafood
Chicken	Eggs

Vegetables:

Acorn squash	Celery
Asparagus	Cucumber
Beetroots	Eggplant
Broccoli	Garlic
Brussels sprouts	Green beans
Butternut squash	Lettuce
Cabbage	Mushrooms
Carrots	Onion
Cauliflower	Pumpkin

Radish

Peppers

Potato (incl. in 2013)

Spinach

Sweet potato

Tomato

Turnip

Zucchini

Fruits:

Apples

Apricots

Bananas

Blackberries

Blueberries

Cherries

Dates **

Grapefruits

Watermelon

Grapes

Kiwi

Melon

Oranges

Pears

Plums

Raspberries

Strawberries

Oil:

Coconut Oil

Ghee

Extra virgin olive oil

Clarified butter

Store Cupboard:

Cashew	Mustard*
Hazelnuts	Coffee
Almonds	Tahini
Pistachio	Curry paste
Walnuts	Chili sauce
Olives	Vinegar*
Coconut/Almond milk	Herbs & Spices
Coconut/Almond flour	Mayonnaise***
Coconut water	

* Check the labels carefully for added sugar

** Limit consuming of dried fruits

*** Check the recipe for homemade mayonnaise at the end of the *Chapter 2. Breakfast Recipes*

4. The golden rules of the diet

Since Whole 30 is not just a diet for losing weight, but a way to switch to a healthy lifestyle, it has several important rules which are strictly obligatory. If you cannot follow them all; then, do not start the program. If you break even just one of them during the clearance, you should start your Whole 30-day challenge from the beginning.

- No any kind of alcohol – even as an additive to food
- No smoking – during the whole month
- No measuring. You are prohibited from weighing or doing any other measurements of your body during the diet. Weigh and measure the waist size on the first day of the program and then at the last one. But not in the middle of the diet
- No calories counting
- Three meals a day is an ideal option, although dried fruits and nuts as snacks are not prohibited. But in reasonable quantities!

Also, a very important thing to remember when doing Whole 30 clearance is to check the label on each product you purchase. A lot of prepackaged goods have added sugar or additives that you might not be aware of. Let's say, bacon, sausages, mayonnaise, etc. You might be shocked at the ingredients included in the foods that you once ate. The levels of sodium, sugar, and additives that have names you cannot even pronounce could be preventing you from maintaining a healthy weight. Becoming conscious about every bite you put in your mouth can help you achieve the healthy weight you desire and stay that way!

5. The Whole Food expected benefits

- Weight loss: Whole 30 will help you to trim down that pesky body fat and give you an excellent body image and attractive physique

- You won't be facing any digestive problems such as stomach bloating, farts or tummy rumblings
- Improving energy potential and physical endurance
- Sleep normalization
- Giving up eating unhealthy snacks
- Normalization of the blood sugar and insulin levels
- Gaining self-confidence
- Reduced occurrences of depression; you will be at peace and your anxiety levels will significantly lower down
- The condition of your skin will vastly improve since you are going for more vegetables and protein while eliminating sugar altogether
- Your hair will be healthier and shinier
- Workout sessions will be more productive

30 days of diet give an opportunity to lose at least of 6-7 kg of weight. Why it happens? Because the diet eliminates processed foods that are often very high in calories derived from added sugar and fat. Eating highly processed and high-calorie foods can quickly make you gain weight especially because such foods lack fiber and are rich in simple sugars, which the body breaks down very fast thus leaving you craving for more after a short period. The high-calorie content coupled with the fact that such foods are digested quickly means that you are likely to eat more of these, which in turn means that you will probably end up with a calorie surplus, thus increasing your chances of gaining weight. Whole 30 foods are satiating due to their dietary fiber, which means that they take a lot of time before they can be eliminated from the body or before the body can signal you to take more food. Besides, they are rich in complex carbohydrates, which are also broken down slowly, so the likelihood of overeating such foods is small. And as such, it is

easy to limit your calorie consumption even if you are not counting calories especially because you end up eating less. The Whole30 foods diet plan does not require any calorie counting, supplements, or complicated meal plans because it is pretty much straight forward; all you have to do is to restrict your intake of processed foods and then start eating mainly whole foods or those that are close to their natural state as possible.

The diet also improves digestion, allows normalizing carbohydrate metabolism and is even able to help with food allergies. The diet with the Whole30 diet includes almost all the groups of foods needed for adequate nutrition. The products of chemical origin (glutamates, amplifiers, and other chemical additives) are excluded from the menu, which also positively affects the state of health.

In addition, it can help a person change his/her food habits and taste preferences. Fans of Whole 30-day diet system assure that the program does not just change eating habits, but significantly affects a person's worldview, an attitude to himself/herself, a health and lifestyle.

6. The Whole Food main difficulties

- *Social pressure*
  If you do not leave alone, get ready to be under the special control of your parents/beloved ones/flatmates. The first week you are going to be attacked with the questions about the diet and be at the center of family jokes – "Gosh, even no cheese?", "It's a hunger strike, not a diet," "You refused even

from chewing gums? Crazy!", and so on. Everyone around will try to feed you. Be strong. And if you have the opportunity to join the program a couple more friends – do it!

- **Food restrictions**
Among the other foods, the diet excludes the use of milk products (except melted butter), which can negatively affect the work of the intestines, the condition of the skin, hair, and nails. For this reason, the Whole30 diet is not recommended for pregnant and lactating women, children, and adolescent girls.

- **Planning**
You need to think in advance (a week or so) about what you will be eating this month. The Whole 30 is not the kind of diet you can go on tomorrow. The preparation – such as doing proper shopping and creating a meal plan is required. Also, this diet on a trip or during some special occasions in your life (like your best friend's birthday) will be particularly challenging.

- **Cooking**
You will find it difficult to finish your whole foods diet if you do not like cooking. You have to be stuck behind the stove at least twice a day. Even people who love cooking after two weeks of the diet can get the treacherous thoughts about "flakes with milk" for dinner. Stay strong! And keep reading the book – our recipes are very easy to make.

7. Side effects of the Whole Food diet

If you have experimented some different diets before joining Whole 30 tribe, then you have most probably seen that there are at least "some" side effects accompanying them. You might be wondering if the diet also has some hidden side effects as well. The good news is that you won't be facing any serious side effects. However, there have been reports of some temporary symptoms which are typical for newcomers. Because of the total sugar elimination, you might experience mood swings, energy fluctuations, sleepiness, and food cravings. The first one-two weeks are usually the toughest. You might experience "carb flu" - you will feel sluggish while your body tries to figure out how to perform without sugar. It will pass.

8. Fantastic tips for the beginners

With all of those out of the way, here are some tips from those who have tried Whole 30-day diet system and want to share their experience to make your Whole 30 journey as pleasant as possible.

- Make up your mind, be aware of all possible difficulties and start when you are fully committed
- Plan, plan, and plan one more time. Carefully plan your first-week meal plan. Then go for the next ones
- Clear out your fridge off all foods that do not match with the diet
- Plan your meals beforehand and do shopping according to it. If you are busy, keep one day aside to

create your meal plan for the rest of the week. Take your lunch to the office

- Cook not something you should cook, but something that will make you happy and keep entertained throughout the month (check our recipes below, there are many decent ones to choose from)
- Have emergency snacks in your bag, car, office, parents' house. This could be some nuts or fruits
- Before starting the Whole30, check out all the coming events... Birthdays, parties... The temptation is great. So keep your food-related socializing events at a minimum
- Involve your friends, family, or housemates – it is always good to go on a diet not alone
- And most importantly, never give up!

9. Life after your Whole Food challenge

After the monthly detox program, the second chapter of your Whole 30 begins – you have to slowly reinstate those products that were eliminated from the diet. Each group of products must be entered separately from the other. You can start with any, but the best is to choose dairy and milk products. So, on the first day after your one-month diet has finished, you start eating dairy products. You eat them throughout the day, and then for four days, you again go back to the Whole30 diet. It is a time to watch your condition carefully.

You have to note any unpleasant symptoms that have not been seen all month, and now they have appeared again after the first day of reintroduction. It can be anything: bloating and diarrhea, itchy skin and queasiness, headache and increased blood pressure. Anything that makes you feel bad.

If you did not notice any unpleasant symptoms within four days after the first "milk day," go on to reinstate into the diet the second group of excluded foods, for example, legumes.

Theoretically, you can return all the excluded products back. However, if you seriously approach to tracking your health after introducing a product group into the diet, you will find that not all of them are consumed by your body normally.

In addition, there are groups of products that you should never consume; like harmful vegetable oils, trans fats, sugar.

Chapter 2: Breakfast Recipes

1. Simple Zucchini Noodles Bowl

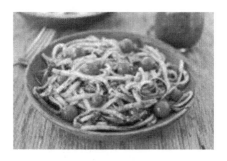

Preparation time: 10 min.	Cooking time: 15 min.	Servings: 2

Ingredients:
- One big zucchini
- Two tablespoons water
- ¼ cup extra virgin olive oil
- ½ avocado
- 2 eggs
- Two tablespoons green onions, chopped
- One garlic clove, chopped
- Two sweet potatoes, peeled and cut
- ½ lemon (juice)
- Salt and black pepper to the taste

Directions:
1. Cut zucchini with the spiralizer, put aside
2. Heat up a pan with two tablespoons olive oil over medium-high heat, add potatoes, occasionally stir and cook for 7-8 minutes.

3. In your food processor, mix avocado with two tablespoons olive oil, garlic, water, salt, and pepper and blend well. After, add a bit of lemon juice.

4. Put zucchini noodles in a bowl, add avocado cream and sweet potatoes and toss.

5. Heat up the pan where you've cooked the potatoes over medium-high heat and cook the eggs until they are done. After, transfer them to zucchini noodles mix.

6. Add more salt and pepper, sprinkle green onions and serve.

Bon Appetite!

Nutrition:

| calories 93 | fat 3 g | fiber 3 g | carbs 11 g | protein4 g |

2. Apple Nut Porridge

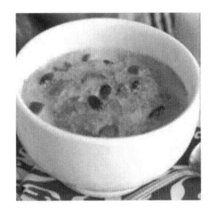

| Preparation time: 15 min | Cooking time: 20 min. | Servings: 4 |

Ingredients:
- 1/2 cup whole raw almonds

- 1/2 cup whole raw cashews
- 1/4 cup raw walnuts
- 1/3 cup unsweetened coconut flakes
- 1 large banana (should be ripe)
- 1 tablespoon ghee (or coconut oil)
- 1 apple, chopped into bite-sized pieces
- 1/8 teaspoon ground nutmeg
- 3/4 cup pure coconut milk
- 2 teaspoon pure vanilla extract
- 2 teaspoon ground cinnamon
- 1/2 cup raisins
- Salt to the taste
- Splash of almond milk (or any of your favorites)

Directions:

1. In a bowl, add the nuts and coconut flakes. Pour water to cover them completely. Add a pinch of salt and cover the bowl. The nuts have to soak at least 7-8 hours or overnight. Once it's done, drain them in a colander until the water runs clear.

2. Put the nuts and coconut flakes into the food processor. Then, add banana (break it into pieces and add to the top of the nuts).

3. Pulse the nuts and banana mixture until it forms a fine nut meal (note – not a paste). Then, remove bowl from food processor and set aside.

4. Add ghee (coconut oil) to a saucepan. After, add the chopped apple and nutmeg and sauté the apples until they begin to soften.

5. Add the coconut milk, cinnamon, vanilla, and raisins. After, add the banana-nut meal mixture. Stir well to mix everything.

6. Bring the porridge to a simmer and cook for 5-7 minutes until it's creamy.

7. Serve the apple porridge with a splash of almond (or any of your favorite) milk.

Bon Appetite!

Nutrition:

calories 180	fat6g	fiber 5,5g	carbs 24g	protein 14g

3. Grain-Free Apple "Oatmeal"

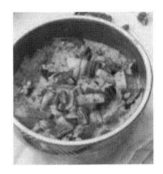

Preparation time: 5 min	Cooking time: 5 min.	Servings: 1

Ingredients:

- 1/2 apple
- 1 date
- 1 tablespoon chia seeds
- 1 tablespoon unsweetened coconut
- 1 tablespoon almonds
- almond butter for the topping
- splash of cashew milk

Directions:
1. Cut the date and the apple into small pieces (not very tiny, though), and place them in a food processor. Add the chia seeds, coconut, and almonds.
2. Pulse mixture until it's grainy and oatmeal-like.
3. Spoon the mixture into a bowl and top with almond butter and milk. Stir together and eat!

Bon Appetite!

Nutrition:

calories 79	fat 5g	fiber 3g	carbs 16g	protein 4g

4. Meatballs Nourishing Salad

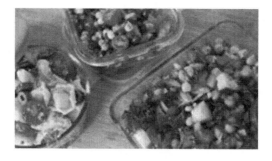

Preparation time: 10 min.	Cooking time: 15 min.	Servings: 4

Ingredients:
- 8 eggs, boiled, peeled and cut into 8 pieces each
- 1 pound breakfast pork sausage
- 3 cups cherry tomatoes, halved
- 2 avocados, chopped
- ¼ cup onion, chopped
- ½ cup cilantro, chopped

- 2 lemons (juice)
- Salt and black pepper to the taste

Directions:
1. Remove casings from sausage, stir the meat and shape into small meatballs.
2. Heat a pan over medium-high heat, after add meatballs, cook until they brown, transfer to a plate and leave them to cool down.
3. In a salad bowl, mix meatballs with eggs, onion, tomatoes, avocado, salt, pepper, cilantro, and lemon juice. Stir and serve right away.

Bon Appetite!

Nutrition:

calories120	fat 4g	fiber 0.5g	carbs 4g	protein 10g

5. Pure Banana Chia Pudding

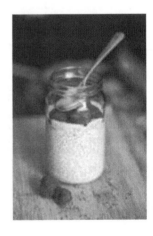

Preparation time: 10 min.	Cooking time: 10 min.	Serving: 6 cups

Ingredients:
- 1 cup water
- 2-1/2 tablespoons chia seeds
- 2 ripe bananas
- 1 cup coconut milk
- 1/2 teaspoon cinnamon
- Salt to the taste

Directions:
1. First, make chia gel.You have to mix the chia seeds and water in a jar with a tight fitting lid. Shake it strongly and set aside for 30 minutes, occasionally shaking to break up any lumps.
2. Second, you should make banana pudding. In the bowl of a food processor or a blender, combine bananas and coconut milk and pulse until smooth.
3. Transfer banana mixture to a bowl and mix in the cinnamon, salt, and chia gel.
4. Store refrigerated and serve cold.

Bon Appetite!

Nutrition:

Calories 118	fat 8 g	fiber 2g	carbs 11g	protein 1g

6. Delicious Zucchini Banana Breakfast

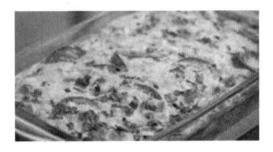

Preparation time: 10 min.	Cooking time: 10 min.	Servings: 1

Ingredients:
- ¾ cup vanilla almond milk
- ¾ cup egg whites
- 1 and ½ tablespoons flax seeds, ground
- One small zucchini, finely grated
- One small ripe banana, peeled and mashed
- ½ teaspoon cinnamon powder

Directions:
1. Grate zucchini. Put it in a bowl, add a mashed banana, stir and leave aside.
2. Heat up a pan over medium heat, add milk and egg whites and mix well.
3. Add flax seeds, stir and cook for 2-3 minutes.
4. Add zucchini mix, stir and cook until the mixture thickens a bit. After, add cinnamon, stir, reduce heat to low and cook for 3 more minutes.
5. Transfer to a bowl and serve right away.

Bon Appetite!

Nutrition:

calories 100	fat 1g	fiber 2g	carbs 0.6g	protein 4g

7. Super Quick Healthy Breakfast Salad

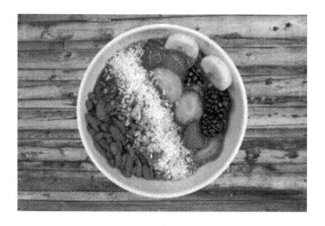

| Preparation time: 5 min. | Cooking time: 0 min. | Servings: 1 |

Ingredients:
- ¼ cup raw cashews
- ¼ cup blueberries (or raspberries)
- One banana
- One tablespoon almond butter
- Cinnamon powder
- Coconut flakes

Directions:
1. Peel and slice bananas. Then, put it in a bowl, mix with cashews and blueberries (or raspberries) and toss.
2. Add cinnamon, a pinch of coconut flakes and almond butter, stir gently and serve right away.

Bon Appetite!
Nutrition:

| calories 90 | fat 0.3g | fiber 1g | carbs 0g | protein 5g |

8. Sweet Potatoes Bowl

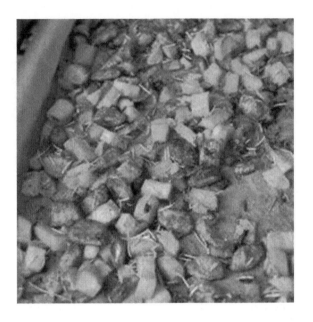

Preparation time:	Cooking time:	Servings:
10 min.	1 hour and 15 min.	1

Ingredients:

- 2 pounds sweet potatoes
- 2 tablespoons water
- ½ pound apples, cored and chopped
- 1 tablespoon ghee
- Salt to the taste

Directions:

1. Put potatoes on a lined baking sheet, introduce in the oven at 400 degrees F and bake for 1 hour.

2. Take potatoes out of the oven, leave them to cool down a bit, peel and mash them in your food processor.

3. Put apples in a pot, add the water, bring to a boil over medium heat, reduce temperature and cook until they are soft.

4. Add this to mashed sweet potatoes, blend again, transfer to a bowl and serve as a breakfast.

Bon Appetite!

Nutrition:

calories 80	fat 1g	fiber 0g	carbs 0g	protein 6g

9. Scrambled Eggs with Salsa Sauce

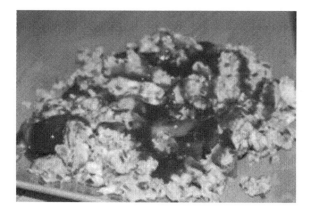

Preparation time: 10 min.	Cooking time: at least 30 min for Salsa sauce. Once it is done, egg cooking takes 5 min.	Servings: 10 to 12

Ingredients:
- 3 medium ripe tomatoes, sliced into small pieces

- 1 bunch green onion, sliced into rounds, white and light green parts only
- 1/2 medium red onion, diced
- 1 bunch cilantro, roughly chopped
- 1 lime
- 1-2 habanero chili (depends on how hot you like it!)
- 2 cloves garlic
- Salt to the taste

Directions:

1. First, you should make salsa sauce*. Combine the tomatoes, green onions, red onions, and cilantro in a bowl. After, mince chili and garlic, so they are almost paste-like, add it to the bowl and stir well. Sprinkle with the salt and squeeze the lime over the top. Toss ingredients together. Chill for at least 30 minutes. It can be in a fridge for up to 5 days.

2. Second, whisk together as many eggs as you need and cook until scrambled.

3. Top with salsa sauce (to the taste) and serve.

* It is a good idea to make a salsa sauce in the evening. The great news is that this sauce is also good with chips, tacos, or any other meal – depends on how strongly you love Salsa.

Bon Appetite!

Nutrition:

Calories 176	fat 7g	fiber 3g	carbs 17g	protein 25

10. Elegant Herb Salmon Frittata

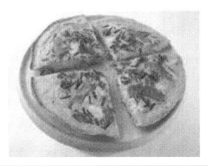

| Preparation time: 10 min. | Cooking time: 30 min. | Serving: 6 |

Ingredients:
- 10 eggs
- 1 small yellow onion, chopped
- 1 and ½ pounds salmon fillets
- 2 tablespoons ghee
- 1 tablespoon dill, chopped
- 1 teaspoon chives, chopped
- 1 teaspoon cilantro, chopped
- 1 tablespoon capers, drained
- 1 tablespoon homemade mayonnaise
- Salt and black pepper to the taste

Directions:
1. Heat up a pan with the ghee over medium high heat, add salmon, salt, and pepper to the taste and cook for 5 minutes.
2. Flip fillets and cook for 3 more minutes and then take off heat.
3. Flake salmon and put in a greased baking dish.
4. In a bowl, mix eggs with pepper, salt, dill, cilantro, capers, and chives and whisk.
5. Pour this over salmon and spread a bit; after, put in the oven at 375 degrees F and bake for 30 minutes.

6. Leave frittata to cool down for a few minutes; after that, put mayonnaise on top.

Bon Appetite!

Nutrition:

calories 100	fat 5g	fiber 3g	carbs 19g	protein 36g

11. Almost Ideal English Breakfast

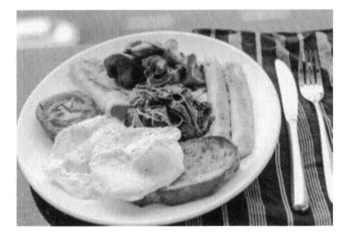

Preparation time: 20 min.	Cooking time: 45 min.	Serving: 2 to 4

Ingredients:
- 2 plum tomatoes
- 2 tablespoons olive oil
- 1/4 teaspoon dried thyme
- 12 medium cremini mushrooms
- 8 small uncooked breakfast link sausages

- 4 large eggs
- Olive oil
- Salt and pepper to the taste
- Toast, for serving (optional)

Directions:

1. Put a rack in the middle of the oven, heat to 425°F. Coat a rimmed baking sheet with olive oil.

2. Halve the tomatoes lengthwise and core the seeds out of them. Place the tomatoes in a bowl, add one tablespoon of oil and half of the thyme, sprinkle with pepper and salt, and toss to combine. Transfer to a baking sheet and arrange cut-side up (reserve the bowl). Roast for 15 minutes.

3. Halve the mushrooms and place in the reserved bowl. When the tomatoes have roasted for 15 minutes, add the rest of olive oil and thyme to the mushrooms, season with salt and pepper, and toss to combine.

4. Remove the baking sheet from your oven; add the sausage and mushrooms, cut-side down. Roast until the sausage is cooked (about 15 minutes).

5. Remove the baking sheet from the oven again. Make four places for the eggs simply using a spatula to push the mushrooms, sausages, and tomatoes aside

6. When it`s done, crack the eggs into those spaces. Sprinkle with pepper and salt. Roast for about 5 minutes for runny yolks or 8 minutes for set yolks. Serve immediately with toast, if using.

Bon Appetite!

Nutrition:

calories 245	fat 8g	fiber 5g	carbs 27g	protein 37g

12. Special Whole 30 Shakshuka

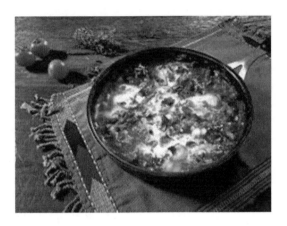

| Preparation time: 10 min. | Cooking time: 30 min. | Servings: 4 |

Ingredients:
- 2 cups brussels sprouts, chopped
- 1 small yellow onion, chopped
- 2 tablespoons extra virgin olive oil
- 1 middle zucchini, grated
- 1 teaspoon cumin
- 4 garlic cloves, minced
- 2 cups baby spinach
- ¼ cup cilantro, chopped
- 4 eggs
- 1 avocado, pitted and sliced
- Salt and black pepper to the taste

Directions:
1. Heat up a pan with the oil over medium heat, add onion, stir and cook for 5 minutes. After, add garlic, stir and cook for 1 minute.

2. Add Brussels sprouts, stir and cook for another 5 minutes.

3. Add salt, pepper, cumin, cilantro, and zucchini, stir and cook for 1 minute more.
4. Add spinach, stir, spread mix, crack eggs on top, introduce everything in the oven and cook at 375 degrees F for 7-8 minutes.
5. Garnish with avocado slices and serve hot.

Bon Appetite!

Nutrition:

calories 160	fat 6g	fiber 2g	carbs 9g	protein 2g

13. Easy Baked Eggs

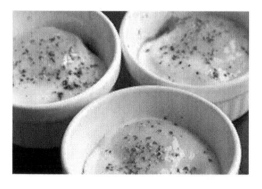

Preparation time: 10 min.	Cooking time: 25 min.	Servings: 4

Ingredients:
- 1 cup water
- 4 eggs
- 1 cup marinara sauce
- Salt and black pepper to the taste

Directions:

1. Heat up a pan with the water over medium-high heat, bring to a simmer, take off heat and pour into a baking dish.
2. Divide marinara sauce in 4 ramekins, crack one egg in each, place ramekins in the baking dish, introduce in the oven and cook at 350 degrees F for 25 minutes.
3. Season baked eggs with salt and pepper and serve hot.

Bon Appetite!

Nutrition:

calories 126	fat 1g	fiber 0.7g	carbs 4g	protein 6g

14. Eggs in a Sweet Potato Nest

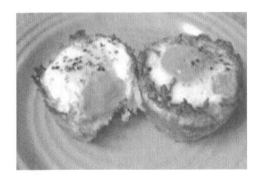

Preparation time: 10 min.	Cooking time: 25 min.	Servings: 5

Ingredients:
- 1 large sweet potato
- 1 sweet apple
- 2,5 tablespoons coconut oil

- 5 large eggs
- Salt to taste
- 3 slices uncooked bacon sliced small
- Balsamic vinegar (optional)
- 1 tablespoon chives (optional)

Directions:

1. Preheat the oven to 350°F. Grease five cups of a jumbo muffin tin with the coconut oil. Set aside.

2. Peel the potato and apple and cut into large pieces (to fit into the food processor). In the bowl of a food processor with the shredder attachment, shred the apple and potato together.

3. In a skillet, heat the two tablespoons coconut oil over medium heat. Add the shredded potato/apple and sauté until softened, about 5 minutes, stirring occasionally. Salt to taste while cooking.

4. Using a 1/2 cup measuring cup, scoop the potatoes out of the skillet and into the greased jumbo muffin cups – it is going to be around 5 cups depending on the size of your potato. Using a small cup, press an indentation into the potatoes, creating a well in the middle and pushing the potatoes up the sides of the muffin cup. This is your nest.

5. Crack one egg into the center of each potato nest. Sprinkle with chives and balsamic vinegar (optional), add salt to taste.

6. Bake in the oven for 17-20 minutes. At this time, you can fry the bacon to desired crispness. Remove from pan with a slotted spoon and drain on a paper towel. Sprinkle bacon bits on top of cooked nests.

Bon Appetite!

Nutrition:

| calories 205 | fat 14g | fiber 1g | carbs 10g | protein 7g |

15. Delicious Breakfast Hash

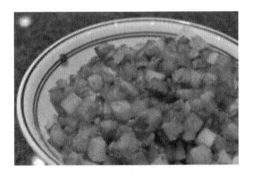

| Preparation time: 10 min. | Cooking time: 25 min. | Servings: 4 |

Ingredients:
- 7 bacon slices, chopped
- 1 celery root, cut into small cubes
- 1 yam, cut into small cubes
- 2 tablespoons ghee
- 4 garlic cloves, finely minced
- 1 small yellow onion, chopped
- 2 tablespoons parsley, finely chopped
- 1 teaspoon smoked paprika
- Salt and pepper to the taste

Directions:
1. Put some water in a pot, add some salt, bring to a boil over medium high heat, add yams, cover, cook for 15 minutes and drain them.

2. Heat up a pan over medium high heat, add bacon pieces, brown them for a few minutes, transfer to a plate and leave aside.

3. Heat up the same pan over medium heat, add onion, stir and cook for 5 minutes.

4. Add celery cubes, stir and cook for 4 minutes more.

5. Add boiled yams, garlic, salt, pepper, paprika, and bacon, stir and cook for 4 minutes more.
6. Divide between plates and serve with parsley sprinkled on top.

Bon Appetite!
Nutrition:

calories 240	fat 2g	fiber 5g	carbs 8g	protein 10g

16. Baked Potato with Avocado Paste

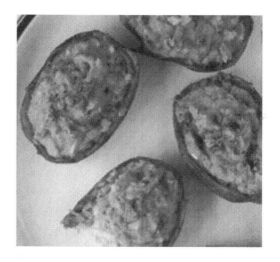

Preparation time: 10 min.	Cooking time: 40 min.	Servings: 3

Ingredients:
- 3 potato, cut into two
- 1 avocado, pitted and sliced
- 1 lime (juice)
- 2 tablespoons extra virgin olive oil

- Garlic powder
- 1 tablespoon chives, chopped
- 1 tablespoon cilantro, chopped
- 1 teaspoon sesame seeds
- Salt, red and black pepper to the taste

Directions:

1. Heat up an oven over medium high heat, add potato slices, season with salt, pepper, garlic powder and drizzle the oil.
2. Bake for 35-40 minutes at 375°F.
3. In the bowl, mix avocado, salt and pepper, red pepper, lime juice, sesame seeds, chives, cilantro, and stir gently.
4. Top each potato slice with avocado paste and serve.

Bon Appetite!

Nutrition:

calories 100	fat 7g	fiber 1g	carbs 5g	protein 10g

17. Avocado Sandwiches with Chicken

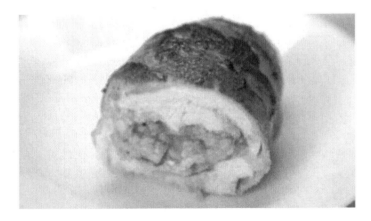

Preparation time: 10 min.	Cooking time: 4 min.	Servings: 2

Ingredients:

- ½ chicken fillet, cut it into 8 thin slices
- 1 avocado, pitted and peeled
- 1 lime (juice)
- 1 tablespoon cilantro
- 1 tablespoon chives
- Salt and black pepper to the taste

Directions:

1. Heat up a pan over medium-high heat, add chicken fillet pieces, brown on all sides, leave for 5 min more to bake and after, transfer to paper towels.
2. Put avocado in your blender, add salt, pepper and lime juice and pulse well. After you have finished, add cilantro and chives and mix well.
3. Spread this mix on two chicken slices, top with the other two pieces and serve with toasts.

Bon Appetite!

Nutrition:

calories 110	fat 5g	fiber 3g	carbs 11g	protein 28g

18. Ruddy Potato Pancakes

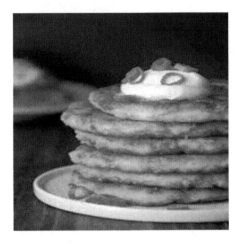

Preparation time: 15 min.	Cooking time: 10 min.	Servings: 4

Ingredients:
- 1 cup zucchini, grated
- 1 cup sweet potato, shredded
- 1 tablespoon coconut flour
- 1 egg, whisked
- ¼ teaspoon cumin, ground
- ½ teaspoon garlic powder
- ½ teaspoon parsley, dried
- 1 tablespoon extra-virgin olive oil
- 1 tablespoon ghee
- Salt and black pepper to the taste
- Herbs – chives, cilantro, dill (additional)
- 2 tablespoons homemade mayonnaise

Directions:
1. In a bowl, combine flour with cumin, salt, pepper, garlic powder, and parsley.

2. In another bowl, mix zucchini with egg and sweet potato and stir.
3. Combine the two mixtures and stir well. Add herbs (if you want) and stir.
4. Heat up a pan with the oil and ghee over medium high heat, shape pancakes from zucchini mix, drop them into the pan, cook until they are gold, flip and cook until they turn golden on the other side as well.
5. Transfer to paper towels, drain grease, divide between plates, top with the mayonnaise and serve hot.

Bon Appetite!

Nutrition:

| calories 122 | fat 8g | fiber 2g | carbs 7g | protein 3g |

19. Almond Pumpkin Porridge

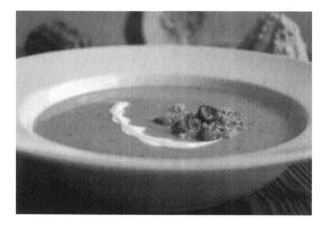

| Preparation time: 10 min. | Cooking time: 10 min. | Serving: 1 |

Ingredients:
- ⅓ cup almond pulp
- 1 tablespoon ground flax or chia seed
- ½ teaspoon ground cinnamon
- 1 cup canned pumpkin
- ⅓ cup almond milk
- 2 teaspoons maple syrup (additional)
- Toppings: nuts, cacao nibs, dried fruit, etc.
- Salt to the taste

Directions:
1. Add the pumpkin, pulp, flax or chia seeds, almond milk, salt, and cinnamon to a small saucepan. Whisk the ingredients together and heat over medium flame till they're starting to bubble.
2. Reduce porridge to a simmer for several minutes, stirring frequently. Remove from heat and drizzle with maple syrup. Sprinkle with toppings as desired, and serve.

Bon Appetite!

Nutrition:

Calories 268	fat 35g	fiber 10g	carbs 17g	protein 16g

20. Tasty Burrito with Lazy Salsa

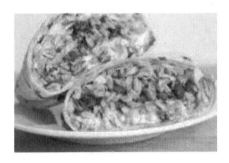

Preparation time: 10 min.	Cooking time: 5 min.	Servings: 1

Ingredients:
- 3 ham slices
- 1 tablespoon spinach leaves, torn
- 1 tablespoon black olives, pitted and chopped
- 1 tablespoon red bell pepper, chopped
- 3 cherry tomatoes, halved
- Olive oil
- 2 eggs, whisked
- 1 tablespoon cilantro, chopped
- Some homemade salsa and guacamole for serving

Directions:
1. Heat up a pan with the oil over medium high heat, add olives, bell pepper, tomatoes and spinach, stir and cook for 3 minutes.
2. Add eggs, stir and cook until they are done.
3. Transfer scrambled eggs to a cutting board, roll ham around them and return to the pan.
4. Heat up the pan for about 2 minutes and transfer burrito to a plate.
5. Serve with salsa, guacamole, and cilantro on top.

Bon Appetite!

Nutrition:

calories 108	fat 2g	fiber 1.4g	carbs 10g	protein 8g

+ How to make gorgeous mayonnaise

Ingredients:
- 1/4 cup + 1 more cup of light olive oil (light, not extra virgin)
- 1 egg
- 1/2 teaspoon mustard powder (check the label for additional sugar)
- 1/2 teaspoon salt
- 1/2 to 1 lemon, juiced

Directions:
1. Make sure that all ingredients (your lemon and egg) are at room temperature.

2. In a food processor (or blender) mix the egg, 1/4 cup of olive oil, mustard powder, and salt.

3. Slowly drizzle 1 cup of olive oil in the food processor while it is running. NOTE: you have to pour that olive oil as slowly as possible. The more slowly you pour, the thicker your mayo will be.

4. After add lemon juice to taste, stirring gently with a spoon to incorporate. NOTE: a lemon goes last.

Enjoy!

Chapter 3: Lunch Recipes

21. Simple Chicken Salad

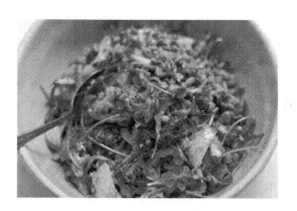

Preparation time: 10 min.	Cooking time: 10 min.	Servings: 4

Ingredients:

- 1 red bell pepper, chopped
- 2 cups chicken meat, already cooked and shredded
- 1 avocado, pitted and chopped
- 2 scallions, finely chopped
- 1 lime (juice)
- ¼ cup cilantro, chopped
- A pinch of cayenne pepper
- ¼ teaspoon smoked paprika
- ¼ teaspoon cumin
- ½ cup nut mix (almond, cashew)
- Salt and black pepper to the taste

Directions:
1. Put avocado pieces in a bowl and mash.
2. In a salad bowl, mix chicken with avocado mash, bell pepper, and scallions and stir gently.
3. Add salt, pepper, lime juice, cilantro, cayenne, cumin, and paprika, and toss to coat.
4. Put nuts on the top and serve.

Bon Appetite!

Nutrition:

calories 120	fat 1g	fiber 2g	carbs 2g	protein 7g

22. Turkey Cauliflower Soup

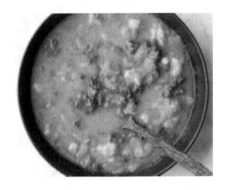

Preparation time: 25 min.	Cooking time: 45 min.	Servings: 4

Ingredients:

- 15 oz. can diced tomatoes
- 1 lb. ground turkey
- 4 shallots, chopped
- 3 carrots, sliced
- 1 bell pepper, cut into pieces

- 5 cups chicken stock
- 1 ½ cup cauliflower, minced
- 4 cups kale, ribs removed, leaves chopped
- 2 tablespoon coconut oil
- Salt and pepper to the taste

Directions:
1. Heat up the saucepan with the coconut oil and add the shallots, carrots, cauliflower, and bell pepper.
2. Cook for about 8-10 min until the vegetables are soft, stirring frequently.
3. Then, add turkey and cook for about 6-8 min.
4. Add the chicken stock, diced tomatoes, and season with salt and pepper.
5. When the soup is boiling, stir in the kale, reduce the heat to low, and let it simmer, covered, for 12-15 min.

Bon Appetite!

Nutrition:

calories 245	fat 20 g	fiber 4	carbs 28 g	protein 37 g

23. Yummy Brothers Burgers

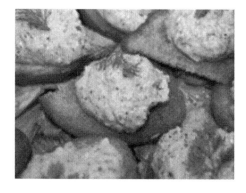

| Preparation time: 10 min. | Cooking time: 10 min. | Servings: 4 |

Ingredients:
- 1 pound turkey meat, ground
- 1 shallot, minced
- 1 jalapeno pepper, minced
- 2 teaspoons lime juice
- Zest from 1 lime
- 1 teaspoon cumin, ground
- 1 teaspoon paprika
- Olive oil
- Salt and black pepper to the taste
- Guacamole for serving

Directions:
1. In a bowl, mix turkey meat with salt, pepper, cumin, paprika, shallot, jalapeno, lime juice and zest and stir well.
2. Shape medium burgers from this combination.
3. Heat up a pan with the olive oil and cook turkey burgers until they are done, flip and cook them on the other side as well.
4. Divide between plates and serve with guacamole on top.

Bon Appetite!
Nutrition:

| calories 200 | fat 12g | fiber 0g | carbs 0g | protein 12g |

24. Salmon with Asparagus Fiesta

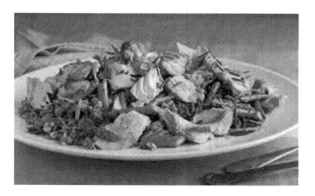

Preparation time: 10 min.	Cooking time: 23 min.	Servings: 4

Ingredients:
- 1 pound asparagus, trimmed
- 1 tablespoon olive oil
- 1 red bell pepper, cut in halves
- 4 ounces smoked salmon
- Sweet paprika
- Garlic powder
- Cayenne pepper
- Salt and black pepper to the taste

Directions:
1. Put asparagus spears and bell pepper on a lined baking sheet.
2. Add salt, pepper, garlic powder, paprika, olive oil, cayenne pepper, toss to coat, introduce in the oven at 390 degrees F and roast for 10-15 minutes.
3. After stir again and bake for 10 minutes more.
4. Leave asparagus and bell pepper to cool down, group 4 asparagus spears, add some bell pepper slices on top and wrap everything with smoked salmon.

5. Repeat with the rest of the asparagus, bell pepper, and salmon, place all bundles on the baking sheet and broil for 5 minutes.
6. Divide between plates and serve.

Bon Appetite!

Nutrition:

| calories 90 | fat 1g | fiber 1g | carbs 1.2g | protein 4g |

25. Super-Easy Tuna Avocado Salad

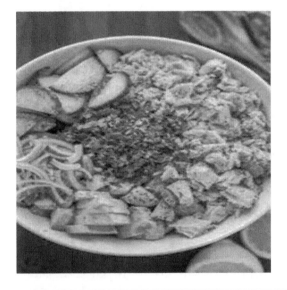

| Preparation time: 30 min. | Cooking time: 0 min. | Servings: 4 |

Ingredients:
- 10 ounces canned tuna (make sure it's soy-free!) in water, drained and flaked

- 1 and ½ avocado, pitted, peeled and roughly mashed
- ½ cup cucumber, chopped
- ½ bell pepper, roughly chopped
- 2 tablespoons red onion, chopped
- ½ cup cilantro, finely chopped
- ½ lime (juice)
- 1 green onion, chopped
- Salt and black pepper to the taste

Directions:
1. In a salad bowl, mix tuna with avocado, cucumber, bell pepper, red onion and green onion.
2. Add salt, pepper, cilantro and lime juice, toss to coat.
3. Leave the salad to cool down in the fridge for 20-40 minutes.

Bon Appetite!

Nutrition:

calories 130	fat 1.5g	fiber 2.4g	carbs 6g	protein 10g

26. Sausage and Kale Sauté

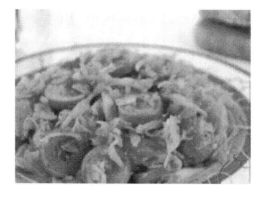

| Preparation time: 10 min. | Cooking time: 15 min. | Serving: 3 to 4 |

Ingredients:
- 1 pound sausage
- 1 bunch kale, chopped into bite size pieces
- 1 onion, diced
- 1/2 red bell pepper, chopped
- Olive oil

Directions:

1. Heat up a large pan and sprinkle with olive oil. After, remove sausage from its casing and brown in a pan.

2. Add the diced onion and continue cooking on medium until the onions are soft.

3. Next, add in kale, mix and cook until it turns bright green(about 5-10 minutes).

4. Remove sausage and kale mixture from the heat, stir in the chopped red bell pepper. Serve warm.

Bon Appetite!

Nutrition:

| calories 184 | fat 4g | fiber 3g | carbs 7g | protein 35g |

27. Simple Herb Salmon

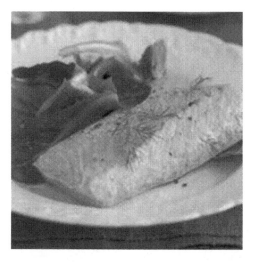

| Preparation time: 10 min. | Cooking time: 25 min. | Servings: 4 |

Ingredients:
- 1 salmon fillet, cut into 4 steaks
- 3 garlic cloves, minced
- 1 yellow onion, chopped
- 2 tablespoons olive oil
- 2 tablespoons tarragon, chopped
- 1 tablespoon dill, chopped
- ¼ cup parsley, chopped
- 1 lemon (juice)
- 1 lemon, sliced
- 1 tablespoon thyme, chopped
- 4 cups water
- Salt and black pepper to the taste

Directions:
1. Heat up a pan with the olive oil, add onion and garlic, stir and cook for 3 minutes.

2. Add salt, pepper, tarragon, parsley, dill, thyme, water, lemon juice and lemon slices, stir and bring to a gentle boil.
3. Add salmon pieces, cook for about 15-18 minutes, and drain it. Better to serve it with a side salad.

Bon Appetite!

Nutrition:

calories 133	fat 3g	fiber 1g	carbs 1g	protein 12g

28. Easy Red Curry Soup

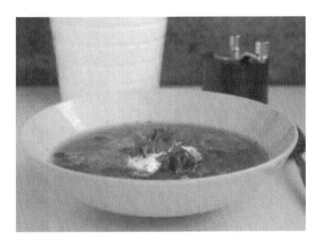

Preparation time: 10 min.	Cooking time: 5 min.	Servings: 1

Ingredients:
- 1/2 cup coconut milk
- 1/2 can fire-roasted diced tomatoes
- 1-2 tablespoons red curry paste (depends on how spicy you want it to be. Check the label for sugar additives!)

- 1/2 tablespoon powdered ginger
- Cooked spaghetti squash
- Leftover cooked veggies (spinach, bell peppers, eggplants, mushrooms)
- Leftover cooked meat (any)

Directions:

1. Add coconut milk, tomatoes, curry paste and ginger to a small saucepan. Stir with a whisk to combine.

2. Cook for 5-6 minutes until the mixture bubbles.

3. Add cooked veggies and meat until heated through. Pour over spaghetti squash to serve.

Bon Appetite!

Nutrition:

Calories 165	fat 10g	fiber 2g	carbs 11g	protein 6g

29. Delightful Mexican Salad

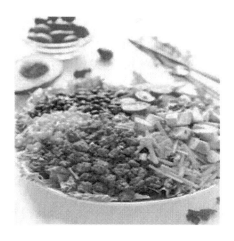

Preparation time: 20 min.	Cooking time: 15 min.	Servings: 4

Ingredients:
- 2 tomatoes, chopped
- 2 avocados, pitted and chopped
- 6 cups romaine lettuce leaves, chopped
- 1 small red onion, chopped
- 2 limes (juice)
- 1 yellow onion, chopped
- 1 pound beef, ground
- 2 garlic cloves, minced
- 1 teaspoon cumin
- 1 tablespoon cilantro, chopped
- 2 teaspoons chili powder
- ½ teaspoon coriander
- Olive oil
- Salt and black pepper to the taste

Directions:
1. Heat up a pan, add olive oil, add yellow onion, stir and cook for 5 minutes.
2. Add garlic, salt, pepper, chili powder, coriander, and cumin, stir and cook for 1 minute.
3. Add beef, stir and cook for 10 minutes and take off heat.
4. In a salad bowl, mix lettuce with avocados, tomatoes, red onion and cilantro and stir.
5. Add beef mix, lime juice, salt, and pepper, toss to coat and serve.

Bon Appetite!

Nutrition:

calories 143	fat 6g	fiber 4g	carbs 12g	protein 6g

30. Stuffed Pepper Soup

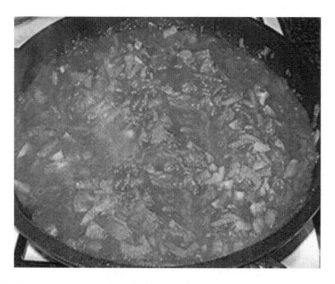

| Preparation time: 15 min. | Cooking time: 45 min. | Servings: 6 |

Ingredients:
- 2 teaspoon coconut oil
- 1 pound ground beef
- 1 onion, diced
- 1 green bell pepper, diced
- 1 14.5 ounces can diced tomatoes
- 1 15 ounces can tomato Sauce (check the label for sugar!)
- 2 cups chicken broth
- 1 teaspoon garlic powder
- Salt and pepper to the taste
- 4 cups cauliflower florets

Directions:
1. Heat coconut oil in a large pot. Add ground beef, onion, and bell pepper; cook breaking up the beef until no pink remains.

2. Stir in tomato sauce, diced tomatoes, and chicken broth. Add garlic powder, salt, and pepper. Bring to a boil; cover and simmer for 20 minutes.
3. Meanwhile, grate your cauliflower (or process in a food processor) to make cauliflower rice.
4. Melt the coconut oil and add the grated cauliflower. Season with salt and pepper. Cook, stirring frequently, for 4-5 minutes or until the cauliflower rice has softened.

Bon Appetite!

Nutrition:

calories 170	fat 3g	fiber 4g	carbs 10g	protein 12g

31. Special Beef with Avocado "Burger"

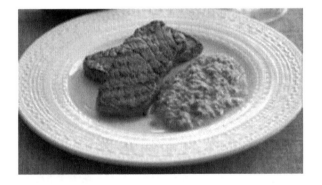

Preparation time: 10 min.	Cooking time: 10 min.	Servings: 7

Ingredients:
- ½ pound bacon, chopped

- 1 and ½ pounds beef, ground
- 6 garlic cloves, minced
- 1 avocado, pitted, peeled and sliced
- Salt and black pepper to the taste

Directions:
1. Put bacon in your food processor and pulse well.
2. In a bowl, mix beef with bacon, garlic, salt, and pepper and stir very well.
3. Shape medium patties from this combination.
4. Heat up a pan over medium high heat, add meat patties, cook for 5 minutes on each side and transfer to plates.
5. Top with avocado slices and serve right away.

Bon Appetite!

Nutrition:

calories 200	fat 5g	fiber 4g	carbs 12g	protein 14g

32. Golden Chicken Egg Muffins

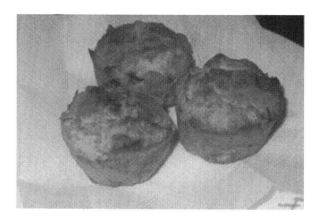

| Preparation time: 10 min. | Cooking time: 40 min. | Servings: 4-6 |

Ingredients:
- 1 pound chicken breasts (boneless, skinless)
- 1/4 cup hot sauce
- 1/4 cup coconut oil
- 12 eggs
- 1/4 cup green onions, sliced
- Salt and pepper

Directions:
1. Preheat oven to 400F. Line a 12-cup muffin tin with papers.

2. Place chicken breasts on a baking sheet and sprinkle salt and pepper on both sides. Bake until cooked through (25-30 minutes). After, remove from oven and set aside to cool slightly. Once the chicken is cool enough, shred and place in a large bowl.

3. In a separate small bowl, stir together hot sauce and coconut oil. Pour half of this mixture over the shredded chicken and stir.

4. In another bowl, put eggs, remaining hot sauce mixture, and green onions. Season with salt and pepper.

5. Fill muffin cups about 12 full with the egg mixture. Top each muffin with about 1/4 cup of chicken.

6. Bake until the eggs tops are golden brown (about 20 minutes). Cool slightly before serving.

7. Reheat after storing in the fridge!

Bon Appetite!

Nutrition:

| calories 380 | fat 20g | fiber 2g | carbs 30g | protein 25g |

33. Sweet Potato and Almonds Bowl

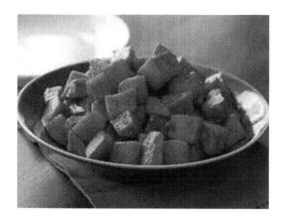

Preparation time: 10 min.	Cooking time: 10 min.	Servings: 3

Ingredients:
- 2 teaspoons olive oil
- 1 sweet potato, cut with a spiralizer
- 3 tablespoons almonds, sliced
- 1 apple, cut with a spiralizer
- 3 cups spinach, torn
- 3 tablespoons raisins
- Salt and pepper

For the vinaigrette:
- 1 teaspoon apple cider vinegar (check the label for sugar additives!)
- 2 tablespoons apple juice
- 1 tablespoon almond butter
- ½ teaspoon ginger, minced
- 1 and ½ teaspoons mustard (also check the label for sugar additives!)
- 1 tablespoon olive oil
- Salt and pepper

Directions:
1. Spread almonds in a pan, introduce in the oven at 350 degrees F and cook for 10 minutes.
2. Heat up a pan with two teaspoons oil, add sweet potato noodles, stir and cook for 5 minutes.
3. Transfer potato noodles to a bowl; add salt, pepper, apple, toasted almonds, spinach, and raisins, and stir.
4. In a heat proof bowl, mix apple juice with cider vinegar and almond butter and stir.
5. Heat up in your microwave for 30 seconds and then mix with one tablespoon olive oil, ginger, salt, and mustard.
6. Whisk this well and add over potato noodles mix.
7. Toss to coat and serve.

Bon Appetite!

Nutrition:

calories 190	fat 2g	fiber 3g	carbs 7g	protein 8

34. Whole 30 Cauliflower Tabbouleh

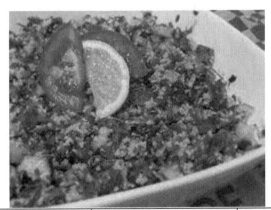

Preparation time: 10 min.	Cooking time: 2 hours	Servings: 4

Ingredients:
- 1/3 cup veggie stock
- 2 tablespoons olive oil
- 6 cups cauliflower florets, grated
- ¼ cup red onion, chopped
- 1 red bell pepper, chopped
- ½ cup kalamata olives, pitted and cut in halves
- 1 teaspoon mint, chopped
- 1 tablespoon parsley, chopped
- ½ lemon (juice)
- Salt and pepper

Directions:
1. Heat up a pan with the olive oil, add grated cauliflower, salt, pepper, and veggies, stir and cook until cauliflower is tender.
2. Transfer cauliflower rice to a bowl and keep in the fridge for 2 hours.
3. Mix cauliflower with olives, onion, bell pepper, salt, pepper, mint, parsley and lemon juice and toss to coat.
4. Serve right away.

Bon Appetite!

Nutrition:

calories 175	fat 12g	fiber 6g	carbs 10g	protein 6g

35. Orange-Avocado Salad

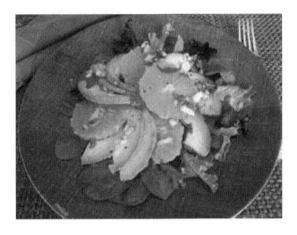

| Preparation time: 10 min. | Cooking time: 0 min. | Servings: 3 |

Ingredients:
- 1 orange, cut into segments
- 2 green onions, chopped
- 1 romaine lettuce head, cut
- 1 avocado, pitted, peeled and chopped
- ¼ cup almonds, roasted and sliced

For the salad dressing:
- 1 teaspoon mustard (check the label for sugar additives!)
- ¼ cup olive oil
- 2 tablespoons balsamic vinegar (check the label for sugar additives!)
- ½ orange (juice)
- Herbs – chive, dill, basil, cilantro, finely chopped (if you wish)
- Salt and black pepper

Directions:

1. In a salad bowl, mix oranges with avocado, lettuce, almonds and green onions.
2. In a small bowl, mix olive oil with vinegar, mustard, orange juice, salt and pepper and whisk well.
3. Add this to salad, after add herbs, mix and serve right away.

Bon Appetite!

Nutrition:

calories 100	fat 0.2g	fiber 2g	carbs 0.4g	protein 4g

36. Special Meatloaf

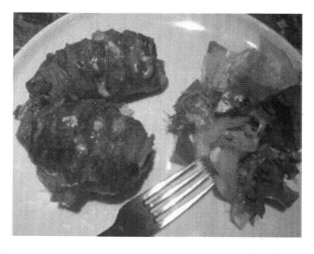

Preparation time: 15 min.	Cooking time: 1 hour	Servings: 8

Ingredients:
- 6 bacon slices
- 2 pounds ground beef
- 1 cup almond flour

- 1/2 onion, finely chopped
- 3 garlic cloves, minced
- 2 eggs
- Salt and pepper

Directions:

1. Preheat oven to 350°F. Line a baking sheet with parchment paper. Fry two slices of bacon until crisp. Crumble and place in a mixing bowl. Reserve the bacon fat!

2. Add almond flour, ground beef, eggs, onion, garlic, the bacon fat, also, salt and pepper and mix well.

3. Place beef mixture on the baking sheet and shape into a loaf form. Top with remaining 4 slices of bacon. Put into oven and cook until cooked through (about 1 hour).

4. Leave it to cool down for 10-15 minutes before slicing and serving.

Bon Appetite!

Nutrition:

calories 175	fat 11g	fiber 0.5g	carbs 6g	protein 14g

37. Spicy Fish Dish

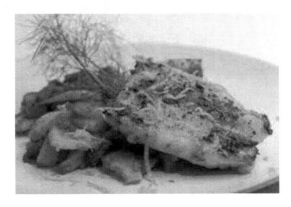

| Preparation time: 10 min. | Cooking time: 15 min. | Servings: 4 |

Ingredients:
- 4 white fish fillets
- ½ lemon (juice)
- 2 fennel bulbs, sliced
- 1 tablespoon coconut oil
- 1 tablespoon olive oil
- Salt and black pepper to the taste

Directions:
1. Season fennel with salt and pepper.
2. Heat up a pan with one tablespoon of the coconut oil, add fennel slices and brown on each side.
3. Reduce heat, cover pan and cook fennel for 10 minutes.
4. Pat dry fish and season with salt and pepper to the taste.
5. Heat up a pan with the olive oil, add fish fillets, cook for 5 minutes, flip and cook for 3 more minutes.
6. Divide fish between plates, add fennel on the side, season with more salt and pepper if needed.
7. Add lemon juice and serve.
Bon Appetite!

Nutrition:

| calories 200 | fat 2g | fiber 4g | carbs 10g | protein 8g |

38. Easy Broccoli Creamy Soup

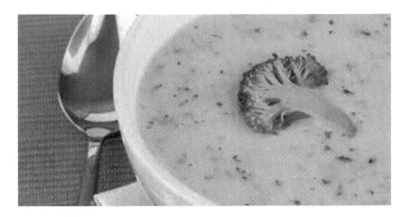

Preparation time: 10 min.	Cooking time: 25 minutes	Servings: 4

Ingredients:
- 4 leeks, white parts chopped
- 2 tablespoons ghee
- 1 yellow onion, chopped
- 1 and ½ pounds broccoli florets, chopped
- 3 shallots, chopped
- ¼ apple, chopped
- 1-quart bone stock
- 1 teaspoon curry powder
- 1 cup coconut milk
- Salt and black pepper to the taste

Directions:

1. Heat up a soup pot with the ghee, add onions, leeks, and shallots, stir and cook for 5 minutes.
2. Add apple, broccoli and stock, salt and pepper, stir and cook for 20 minutes. Then add more salt and pepper, curry powder, stir and transfer to your blender.

3. Pulse well until it is creamy, add coconut milk, pulse again and return soup to the pot.
4. Bring soup to a boil, take off heat and divide into bowls.

Bon Appetite!

Nutrition:

calories 150	fat 8g	fiber 1g	carbs 10g	protein 7g

39. Delightful Chili

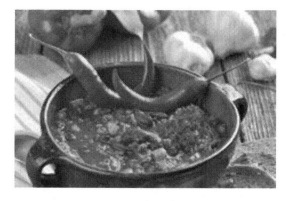

Preparation time: 30 min.	Cooking time: 1 hour	Servings: 4

Ingredients:

- 2 pounds sirloin steak, cut into bite-sized pieces
- 1 big yellow onion, chopped
- 1 Jalapeño chili, minced
- 2 cloves garlic, minced
- 4 slices bacon

- 1 tablespoon chili powder
- 2 teaspoons smoked paprika
- 1 teaspoon cumin
- 14 ounces diced tomatoes, fire-roasted
- 8 ounces tomato sauce (check the label for sugar additives!)
- 1 cup chicken broth
- Herbs – dill, cilantro, basil (if you wish)
- Salt and pepper

Directions:
1. Heat a large pot over medium heat. Add bacon and cook until crisp. Remove bacon to a paper-towel lined plate, but leave a little bit of remaining fat in the pot.
2. Roast sirloin steak for 2 min. each side.
3. Add onion and jalapeno; cook, stirring occasionally until they have softened.
4. Add garlic and cook another 30 seconds, until the garlic is fragrant.
5.Add smoked paprika, chili powder, cumin, and stir. Add salt and pepper. Stir well again.
6. Add in tomatoes, chicken broth, and tomato sauce, and stir well.
7. Bring to a boil, cover, and leave to simmer for about an hour.
8. Put herbs on the top of each plate and serve hot!

Bon Appetite!

Nutrition:

calories 226	fat 8g	fiber 6.3g	carbs 21g	protein 20g

40. Mushrooms Soup with Chicken

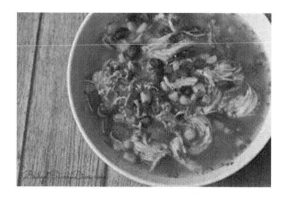

Preparation time: 10 min.	Cooking time: 30 min.	Servings: 6

Ingredients:
- 1 bunch kale, chopped
- 2 quarts chicken stock
- 1 cup chicken, shredded
- 3 carrots, chopped
- 1 cup button mushrooms, sliced
- Salt and black pepper to the taste

Directions:
1. Reserve 2 cups stock and heat up the rest over medium heat.
2. Pour reserved stock in a blender, add kale, pulse a few times and pour this overheated soup.
3. Add chicken, mushrooms, and carrots, stir and cook for 30 minutes.
4. Add salt and pepper, cook for 4 minutes more and ladle into soup bowls.

Bon Appetite!

Nutrition:

calories 180	fat 7g	fiber 2g	carbs 10g	protein 5g

Chapter 4: Side Dish Recipes

41. Fantastic Brussels Sprouts

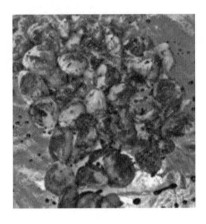

Preparation time: 10 min.	Cooking time: 30 min.	Servings: 4

Ingredients:
- 1 pound brussels sprouts
- 1 tablespoon olive oil
- 1/4 cup lemon juice
- 1/2 cup water
- ¼ cup sun dried tomatoes in oil, drained and chopped
- 1 teaspoon mustard (check the label for sugar additives)
- 1 teaspoon arrowroot + 1 tablespoon cold water
- Salt and pepper

Directions:
1. Prepare Brussels sprouts – cut off the bottom and chop each one in half.

2. Preheat oven to 400 F.

3. Place Brussels sprouts on the cookie sheet lined with foil. On the top, generously pour olive oil. Add pepper and salt. Toss.

5. Roast for about 20 min.

4. Meanwhile, place a skillet over medium high heat. Add water, lemon juice, tomatoes and bring to a boil. After, add arrowroot and water mixture and stir quickly as it will seize up! Add mustard and season with salt and pepper. Add a little extra water in case sauce is too thick.

5. Place cooked brussels sprouts in a bowl and then toss with about ¼ cup of sauce.

Bon Appetite!

Nutrition:

calories 88	fat 4.5g	fiber 4g	carbs 11.7g	protein 4.1g

42. Sweet Potato Salad

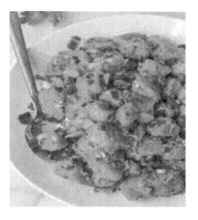

Preparation time: 10 min.	Cooking time: 40 min.	Servings: 4

Ingredients:
- 4 sweet potatoes, cubed
- Olive oil
- ¼ cup coconut, unsweetened and shredded
- 1/3 cup macadamia nuts, chopped
- 2 cups pineapple, chopped
- 1 cup coconut yogurt
- 1/3 cup almond milk

Directions:
1. Drizzle the oil over potato cubes, toss to coat, spread them on a baking sheet and bake in the oven at 350 degrees F for 40 minutes.
2. Transfer potatoes to a bowl, add nuts, coconut, and pineapple and toss to coat.
3. Add almond milk and coconut milk, stir to coat and serve.

Bon Appetite!

Nutrition:

calories 100	fat 11g	fiber 0.3g	carbs 17g	protein 4g

43. Super-Quick Pineapple Salsa

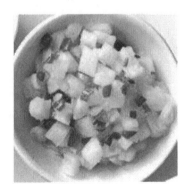

Preparation time: 15 min.	Cooking time: 15 min.	Servings: 6

Ingredients:
- 2 cups diced fresh pineapple
- 1/4 cup diced jalapeno pepper
- 1 cup diced red onion
- 1/4 cup cilantro
- 2 tablespoons lime juice
- Salt and pepper

Directions:
1. In a small bowl, place all the ingredients and mix well.
2. Add salt, pepper and lime juice.Mix again.
2. Cover and refrigerate until serving.

Bon Appetite!

Nutrition:

calories 30	fat 2gg	fiber 0.4g	carbs 8g	protein 3g

44. Roasted Garlic Potatoes

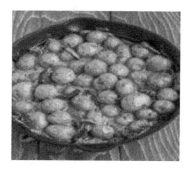

Preparation time: 10 min.	Cooking time: 30 min.	Servings: 4

Ingredients:
- 8 sweet potatoes, chopped
- 1 teaspoon turmeric
- 3 tablespoons coconut oil
- ½ teaspoon ginger, ground
- ½ teaspoon cloves
- 1 cup parsley, chopped
- 1 lemon (juice)
- 1 garlic clove, minced
- ¾ cup olive oil
- 2 tablespoons tahini
- Salt and black pepper to the taste

Directions:
1. In a bowl, mix potatoes with coconut oil, salt, and pepper, toss to coat and spread on a lined baking sheet.
2. Introduce in the oven at 400 degrees F and bake for 30 minutes, stirring them after 20 minutes have passed.
3. In a bowl, mix parsley with garlic, lemon juice, olive oil, salt, and tahini. Whisk well.
4. Take potatoes out of the oven, transfer to a bowl, drizzle the sauce over them, toss to coat well and serve as a side dish right away.

Bon Appetite!

Nutrition:

calories 230	fat 3g	fiber 6g	carbs 9g	protein 10g

45. Healthy Green Salad

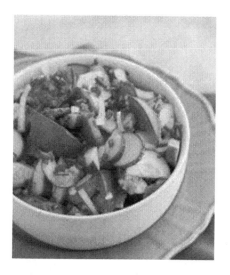

Preparation time: 10 min.	Cooking time: 5 min.	Servings: 4

Ingredients:
- 6 large tomatoes, sliced
- 1 red onion, chopped
- 1 large cucumber, sliced
- 2 large red bell peppers, sliced
- 1/2 cup sliced olives
- 1/3 cup chopped pepperoni

For the dressing:
- 1/4 cup olive oil
- 1/4 cup balsamic vinegar (check the label for sugar additives)
- 1/2 teaspoon minced garlic
- 1 tablespoon chopped fresh basil
- 1 tablespoon chopped fresh oregano
- 1 tablespoon chopped fresh cilantro
- 1 tablespoon chopped fresh dill

Directions:
1. In a large bowl, mix the tomato, onion, cucumber, pepper, olives, and pepperoni.
2. In a small bowl, mix all the ingredients for the dressing
3. Pour the dressing over the fresh vegetables and serve immediately.

Bon Appetite!

Nutrition:

calories 103	fat 7g	fiber 1g	carbs 3g	protein 0g

46. Delicious Potato with Bacon

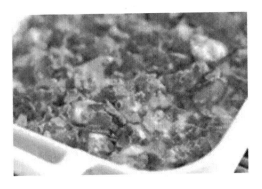

Preparation time: 10 min.	Cooking time: 30 min.	Servings: 4

Ingredients:
- 8 bacon slices, chopped
- 1 and ½ pounds potatoes, cut into medium rounds
- 2 garlic cloves, minced
- 7 sage leaves
- 1 tablespoon rosemary, chopped
- Salt and black pepper to the taste

Directions:
1. Put some water into a pot, add salt and potatoes, bring to a boil over medium-high heat, cook for 7 minutes, drain and rinse them.
2. Heat up a pan over medium-high heat; add bacon, stir, brown for 10 minutes and transfer to a bowl.
3. Add potatoes to the pan, cook for 20 minutes stirring occasionally, and season with salt and pepper. After that, add bacon, rosemary, garlic, and sage, stir and cook for a few more minutes.
4. Mix and serve.

Bon Appetite!

Nutrition:

calories 300	fat 12g	fiber 4g	carbs 20g	protein 4g

47. Bacon with Thyme Mashed Cauliflower

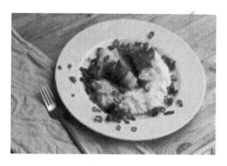

Preparation time: 15 min.	Cooking time: 20 min.	Servings: 6

Ingredients:
- 2 lbs. cauliflower florets
- 2 garlic cloves
- 6 bacon slices

- 2 tablespoons ghee or grass-fed butter
- 1 teaspoon thyme, chopped
- 1 tablespoon ghee
- Salt and pepper

Directions:
1. In the water boil garlic and cauliflower until tender.
2. Meanwhile, cook bacon to desired crispness.
3. Pulse bacon in a food processor until small bits are created.
4. Add cooked cauliflower to a food processor along with ghee and process until smooth.

Bon Appetite!

Nutrition:

calories 80	fat 5 g	fiber 3 g	carbs 7 g	protein 2 g

48. Amazingly Simple Potato Salad

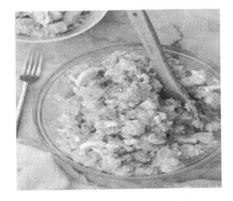

Preparation time: 10 min.	Cooking time: 40 min.	Servings: 4

Ingredients:
- 4 sweet potatoes, cubed
- 1 and ½ cups cranberries, frozen
- 1 tablespoon extra-virgin olive oil
- ½ cup coconut milk yogurt
- ¼ cup pecans, crushed

Directions:
1. Spread potato cubes on a baking sheet, drizzle the oil, toss to coat and bake at 350 degrees F for 45 minutes.
2. Heat up a pan over medium heat, add cranberries and cook until they become a thick sauce.
3. Transfer cranberries to a bowl, add pecans and yogurt and stir well.
4. Put potatoes in a salad bowl, add cranberries sauce, toss to coat well and serve cold as a side dish.

Bon Appetite!

Nutrition:

calories 223	fat 8g	fiber 5.5g	carbs 20g	protein 5g

49. Hot Egg with Squash Soufflé

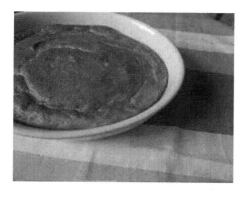

Preparation time: 10 min.	Cooking time: 1 hour	Servings: 4

Ingredients:
- 1 butternut squash
- 4 egg whites
- 4 egg yolks
- ½ cup coconut milk
- Salt and black pepper to the taste

Directions:

1. Wash one butternut squash (do not need to cut).
2. Preheat your oven at 350F.
3. Bake squash in the oven for 17-20 min. Take it out, leave aside to cool down and scoop flesh into the blender.
2. Add salt, pepper, egg yolks and coconut milk and blend well.
3. In a bowl, beat egg whites.
4. Transfer squash mixture to a bowl, add egg whites and stir.
5. Grease the baking dish and transfer this to it. Bake in the oven at 350 degrees F for 40 minutes.
6. Serve hot as a side dish.

Bon Appetite!

Nutrition:

calories 203	fat 13g	fiber 2g	carbs 16g	protein 4g

50. Spicy Golden Brown Potato Chips

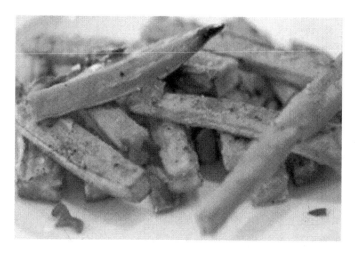

Preparation time: 20 min.	Cooking time: 25 min.	Servings: 3

Ingredients:
- 3 sweet potatoes, cut into fry shapes
- 3 tablespoons olive oil
- 3 tablespoons arrowroot starch
- 1 teaspoon ground coriander
- 1/2 teaspoon fennel seed
- 1/2 teaspoon dried oregano
- 1/2 teaspoon crushed red pepper flakes
- 1/2 teaspoon salt
- ½ cup homemade mayonnaise

Directions:
1. Leave chopped sweet potatoes to soak in water for at least an hour. This pulls out some of the starch in the potatoes and helps them to crisp up. After dry the potatoes.
2. Preheat the oven to 400 degrees and spray a baking sheet with olive oil.
3. Place the potatoes in the bowl, add olive oil and toss. Add arrowroot starch and toss again.

4. Arrange the potatoes on the prepared baking sheet. The potato fries should be in a single layer, not touching each other at all.

5. In a small bowl, mix together the coriander, fennel, oregano, red pepper flakes, and salt. Sprinkle the seasonings over the potatoes.

6. Place the potatoes in the oven and bake it for 30. Watch closely as the time might vary depending on how thick or thin potato pieces are.

7. Serve with homemade mayonnaise.

Bon Appetite!

Nutrition:

calories 272	fat 14 g	fiber 4 g	carbs 35 g	protein 2 g

51. Tuscan Chicken Spaghetti Squash

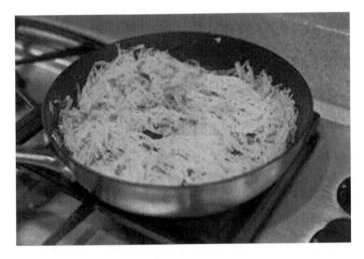

Preparation time: 15 min.	Cooking time: 1 hour	Servings: 4-6

Ingredients:
- 1 medium spaghetti squash
- 2½ cups shredded chicken
- ⅔ c sun dried-tomatoes packed in oil (drained)
- ½ cup fresh basil, chopped
- 3 eggs
- 1 tablespoon full-fat coconut milk

Directions:
1. Preheat oven to 375 degrees. Cut the squash horizontally and scoop out the seeds. Pour 2 inches of water in a baking dish, then place the cut side of the squash in the pan and cook for 35-45 minutes. After, shred the softened squash with a fork to create spaghetti-looking noodles.
2. In a large bowl, add the shredded squash, chicken, tomatoes, and basil.
3. In a separate bowl, whisk the eggs and coconut milk
4. Pour the egg mixture into the spaghetti squash and mix well. Then pour the entire mixture into a baking dish and bake for 30 minutes.
5. You can serve it hot as well as cold.

Bon Appetite!

Nutrition:

calories 162	fat 8g	fiber 2g	carbs 16g	protein 4g

52. Spinach with Avocado "Zoodles"

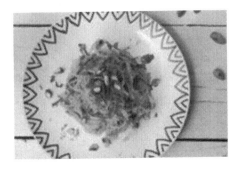

Preparation time: 10 min.	Cooking time: 5 min.	Servings: 4

Ingredients:
- 3 zucchinis, cut with a spiralizer
- 1 cup fresh basil, chopped
- ½ tablespoon olive oil
- 1 cup spinach, finely chopped
- 2 garlic clove, minced
- 1 avocado pitted and peeled
- 1/3 cup cashews, roasted
- 1 lemon (juice and zest)
- Salt and pepper

Directions:
1. Put spinach with basil, avocado, cashews, salt, lemon zest and lemon juice in the food processor, and blend well.
2. Heat up a pan with the oil over medium high heat, add zucchini noodles (I call them zoodles), stir and cook for 5 minutes.
3. Add spinach and avocado sauce, stir, cook for 1 minute more and transfer to plates.

Bon Appetite!

Nutrition:

calories 200	fat 4g	fiber 2g	carbs 10g	protein 8,5g

53. Mushrooms with Green Beans Side Dish

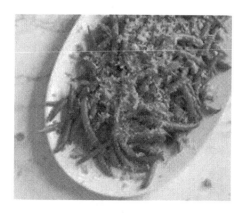

Preparation time: 10 min.	Cooking time: 10 min.	Servings: 4

Ingredients:
- 1 pound green beans
- 2 cups cremini mushrooms, chopped
- 1 tablespoon avocado oil
- ½ cup almonds, toasted and sliced
- 1 garlic clove, minced
- Salt and black pepper to the taste

Directions:
1. Heat up a pan with the avocado oil over medium-high heat, add the garlic clove, stir and cook for 1 minute. Add mushrooms, cook for 10 more minutes.
2. Add green beans, salt, and pepper, stir together and cook for 10 minutes.
3. Add almonds, stir, take off heat, divide between plates and serve.

Bon Appetite!

Nutrition:

calories 140	fat 2g	fiber 6g	carbs 12g	protein 6g

54. Thai Shrimp Salad

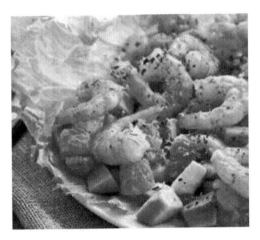

Preparation time: 15 min.	Cooking time: 10 min.	Servings: 2

Ingredients:

- 6 cups shredded romaine lettuce
- 1 red bell pepper, diced
- ½ cup matchstick carrots
- ¼ cup fresh cilantro
- ¾ cup cucumbers, diced
- ⅓ cup cashews, raw
- ½ pound cocktail shrimp, thawed and peeled

Almond Dressing

- 2 tablespoons almond butter
- ⅛ cup olive oil
- 1 teaspoon coconut aminos
- ½ teaspoon rice vinegar (check the label for sugar additives)
- ½ teaspoon sesame oil
- 1 tablespoon lime juice
- 1½ teaspoons water

Directions:
1. Add to a large bowl pepper, lettuce, carrot, cucumbers, and cilantro. Toss well
2. Add the cocktail shrimps. Mix.
3. In another bowl, mix the almond dressing ingredients well and drizzle over the salad.
4. Top the salad with cashews.

Bon Appetite!

Nutrition:

calories 76	fat 2g	fiber 3g	carbs 9g	protein 1,5g

55. Tasty Onion with Mushroom Side Dish

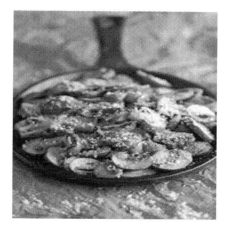

Preparation time: 10 min.	Cooking time: 20 min.	Servings: 4

Ingredients:
- 4 cups oyster mushrooms
- 1 cup onion, chopped

- 2 tablespoons ghee
- Garlic powder
- A handful tarragon, chopped
- 2 tablespoons chives, chopped
- 1 tablespoon cilantro, chopped
- Salt and black pepper to the taste

Directions:
1. Heat up a pan with the ghee, add onions, cook 2-3 minutes, stirring frequently.
2. Add mushrooms, salt, pepper and garlic powder, stir, reduce heat to medium and cook for 20 minutes.
3. Sprinkle tarragon and chives, stir, take off heat and divide between plates.

Bon Appetite!

Nutrition:

calories 200	fat 12g	fiber 7g	carbs 29g	protein 14g

56. French Celeriac Fries

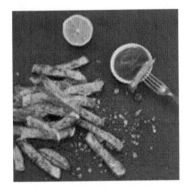

Preparation time: 10 min.	Cooking time: 25 min.	Servings: 4

Ingredients:
- 1 tablespoon olive oil
- 1 celeriac, cut in thin fries
- ½ teaspoon paprika
- Salt and black pepper to the taste
- ½ cup homemade mayonnaise

Directions:
1. In a bowl, mix celeriac fries with salt, pepper, paprika, and oil and toss to coat well.
2. Spread this on a lined baking sheet and bake in the oven at 400 degrees F for 25 minutes, shaking from time to time the baking sheet.
3. Use homemade mayonnaise like sauce. Serve right away as a side dish!

Bon Appetite!

Nutrition:

calories 50	fat 4g	fiber 1g	carbs 5g	protein 1g

57. Carrot and Garlic Salad

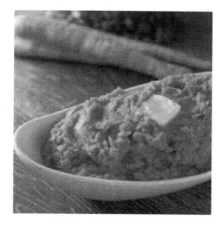

Preparation time: 10 min.	Cooking time: 1 hour	Servings: 3

Ingredients:
- 5 large carrots
- one tablespoon ghee
- 2 garlic cloves, minced
- 2 tablespoons homemade mayonnaise
- Salt and black pepper to the taste

Directions:
1. Cut each carrot into 2-3 pieces and boil into a saucepot until it's soft (45-50 minutes). When it is ready, put aside for 15-20 minutes to cool down.
2. Grade the carrots, add garlic, salt, pepper, and ghee and stir everything well. Add mayonnaise and again stir.
3. Leave it in the fridge to cool down for 20-30 min.

Bon Appetite!

Nutrition:

calories 86	fat 4g	fiber 3g	carbs 15g	protein 0g

58. Soft Cauliflower Puree

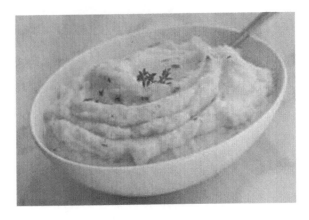

Preparation time: 10 min.	Cooking time: 20 min.	Servings: 4

Ingredients:
- 6 cups cauliflower florets
- 2 tablespoons ghee (or olive oil)
- Salt and black pepper to the taste

Directions:
1. Boil water in a pot, add some salt, add cauliflower and cook for 15 minutes.
2. After, drain and reserve 1 cup cooking liquid.
3. In your blender, mix cauliflower with reserved cooking liquid, salt, and pepper and blend well.
4. Add ghee (or olive oil), mix again and divide among plates.

Bon Appetite!

Nutrition:

calories 91	fat 4g	fiber 3g	carbs 8g	protein 4g

59. Creamy Spinach

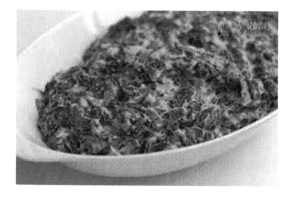

| Preparation time: 10 min. | Cooking time: 5 min. | Servings: 4 |

Ingredients:

- ½ cup homemade mayonnaise
- 6 cups spinach
- 2 tablespoons chicken stock
- ½ teaspoon garlic, minced
- 1 tablespoon lime juice
- ¼ teaspoon cumin
- ¼ teaspoon chipotle powder
- Salt and pepper to the taste

Directions:

1. Put in a bowl mayonnaise, stock, garlic, lime juice, chipotle powder, cumin, and salt and stir well.
2. Heat up a pan, add mixture, stir and cook for 5 minutes.
3. Add spinach, stir and cook for 5 minutes more.
4. Take off heat, divide between plates and serve as a side dish.

Bon Appetite!

Nutrition:

| calories 147 | fat 8g | fiber 3g | carbs 11g | protein 5g |

60. Simple Sautéed Kale with Garlic

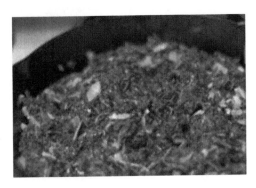

Preparation time: 5 min.	Cooking time: 5 min.	Servings: 4

Ingredients:

- 6 cups kale, chopped
- 2 tablespoons ghee (or olive oil)
- 1 tablespoon lemon juice
- 1-2 garlic cloves, finely minced

Directions:

1. Wash the kale, then tear the leaves off the stem and shred into small, bite-sized pieces.

2. Heat ghee (or olive oil) in a large saucepan and add the kale.

3. Add the lemon juice and garlic. Stir. Cook for about 5 minutes

4. Serve immediately or let cool and refrigerate to store.

Bon Appetite!

Nutrition:

calories 43	fat 0g	fiber 2g	carbs 9g	protein 0g

Chapter 5: Snacks and Appetizer Recipes

61. Flaxseed Crackers

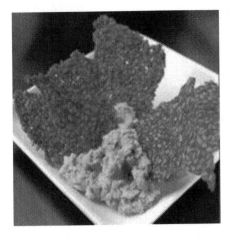

| Preparation time: look the recipe | Cooking time: 1 hour | Servings: 1 |

Ingredients:
- 1 cup flax seeds
- 2 cups water
- ½ teaspoon salt
- 2 teaspoons fresh rosemary, chopped
- 1 teaspoon lemon juice

Directions:
1. In a bowl , mix water and flaxseeds and let sit for at least one hour or even overnight. After the mixture has set, the water in the mixture should form a gel-like consistency.
2. Add the salt, rosemary, and lemon juice.

3. Line a baking sheet with parchment paper.
4. Pour the mixture in a thin layer on a baking sheet. Now you need to dehydrate it for 15 hours (at 115 F). Make sure, that the bottom is dry and the flaxseed is crispy.
5. If you are making the crackers in the oven, preheat to 325 degrees and bake for 1 hour.
6. Once the flaxseed crackers are in consistency, simply break off the sheet into small-bite sized portions.

Bon Appetite!

Nutrition:

calories 45	fat 0g	fiber 1g	carbs 5g	protein 0g

62. Fried Eggplant Medallions

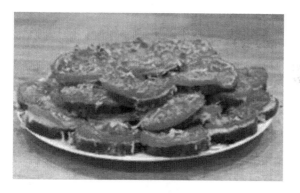

Preparation time: 15 min.	Cooking time: 15 min.	Servings: 2

Ingredients:
- 2 eggplants, cut into slices
- 2 tomatoes, cut into slices
- 1 garlic clove, finely minced
- 1 teaspoon cilantro, finely minced

- 1 teaspoon dill, finely minced
- 2 tablespoons homemade mayonnaise
- 1 tablespoon olive oil
- Salt and pepper

Directions:
1. In the bowl, put eggplants slices, add salt and pepper and stir gently. Leave for 10-15 minutes.
2. After that, heat up a pan, add olive oil, put eggplants slices in and fry until both sides are brown.
3. Transfer to the plate to cool down.
4. In a small bowl, mix mayonnaise, garlic, cilantro, and dill. Smear eggplants slices with mayonnaise mixture.
5. Put tomato slices on top of each eggplant slices. Leave it to cool in the fridge for 30 minutes.

Bon Appetite!

Nutrition:

calories 37	fat 2g	fiber 1g	carbs 9g	protein 0g

63. Egg and Cucumber Snack

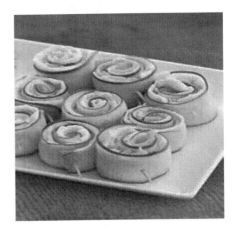

| Preparation time: 10 min. | Cooking time: 7 min. | Servings: 1 |

Ingredients:
- 2 eggs
- 1 cucumber, cut into medium slices
- 1 tablespoon dill, chopped
- ¼ teaspoon paprika
- Salt and black pepper

Directions:
1. Put some water in a pot, add eggs, bring to a boil over medium heat, cook for 7 minutes, drain and transfer to a bowl filled with cold water.
2. Cool down eggs, peel them and slice them.
3. Arrange cucumber slices on a plate, add egg slices on top, sprinkle salt, pepper, and paprika and serve with dill on top.

Bon Appetite!

Nutrition:

| calories 170 | fat 5g | fiber 1g | carbs 2g | protein 14g |

64. Fried Plantains with Mango Salsa

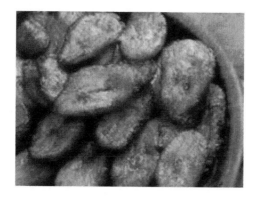

Preparation time: 10 min.	Cooking time: 10 min.	Servings: 4

Ingredients:
- 4 green plantains, peeled and each cut into 2-inch pieces
- 4 cups coconut oil
- Salt

For the mango salsa:
- 1 avocado, pitted, peeled and cubed
- 2 cups mango, cubed
- ¼ cup cilantro, chopped
- ½ cup red onion, chopped
- 2 tablespoons olive oil
- Salt and black pepper to the taste
- 1 lime (juice)
- A pinch of red pepper flakes

Directions:
1. Heat up a pan with the coconut oil over medium high heat, add plantain pieces, fry for 5 minutes on both sides, and transfer to paper towels.
2. Place plantains on a sheet of parchment paper, add another one over them and press with a meat pounder.
3. Heat up the pan with the oil again over medium high heat, add plantain patties, cook them for 5 minutes more, drain on paper towels and arrange on a platter.
4. In a bowl, mix avocado with mango, onion, and cilantro.
5. Add olive oil, salt, pepper and pepper flakes, toss to coat and serve your plantains with the salsa on the side.

Bon Appetite!

Nutrition:

calories 200	fat 3g	fiber 9g	carbs 8g	protein 12g

65. Savory Stuffed Dates

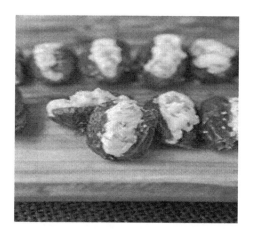

| Preparation time: 10 min. | Cooking time: 0 min. | Servings: 1 |

Ingredients:
- 2 medjool dates, cut on one side
- 5 pistachios, raw and chopped
- 1 teaspoon coconut, shredded

Directions:
1. In a bowl, mix chopped pistachios with coconut and stir very well.
2. Stuff each date with this mix and serve them right away.

Bon Appetite!

Nutrition:

| calories 60 | fat 1g | fiber 0g | carbs 0.2g | protein 1g |

66. Marvelous Energy Snacks

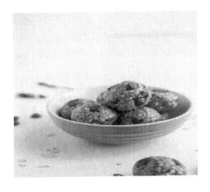

Preparation time: 10 min.	Cooking time: 12 min.	Servings: 8

Ingredients:
- 1 cup dried fruits
- 1 cup dates, pitted and dried
- 1 cup nuts mix (cashew, walnuts)

Directions:
1. Spread nuts on a lined baking sheet and roast in the oven at 350 degrees F for 15 minutes. After nuts have cooled down, put them in the food processor.
2. Add dried fruit and dates and blend well. After, shake processor a bit and pulse again for 2 minutes.
3. Spread this on a wax paper, press dough well into a square, cover and keep in the fridge for 1 hour.
4. Cut into 8 bars and serve as a snack
.

Bon Appetite!

Nutrition:

calories 200	fat 7g	fiber 4g	carbs 41g	protein 4g

67. Great Chicken Appetizer

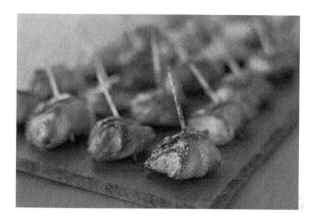

Preparation time: 10 min.	Cooking time: 20 min.	Servings: 6

Ingredients:
- 2 chicken breast, cut into thin strips
- 4 tablespoons arrowroot powder
- 1 cup almond flour
- ½ cup coconut, shredded
- 1 teaspoon mustard powder
- 1 teaspoon garlic powder
- 1 teaspoon paprika
- 2 tablespoons sesame seeds
- A pinch of cayenne pepper
- 3 tablespoons olive oil
- 2 eggs
- Salt and black pepper to the taste

For the dip:
- 1 lemon (zest and juice)
- 4 mint sprigs, chopped
- 1 garlic clove, minced
- Salt and black pepper to the taste

Directions:
1. In a bowl whisk eggs with a pinch of salt.
2. In a second bowl, whisk flour with coconut, arrowroot powder, paprika, mustard, salt, pepper, cayenne and sesame seeds and stir.
3. Dip chicken in egg and then in the almond mix, spread strips on a lined baking sheet, drizzle the olive oil all over them and bake in the oven at 400 degrees F for 20 minutes.
4. In a bowl, mix mint, lemon juice, lemon zest, garlic clove, salt and pepper and whisk well. Ready!

Bon Appetite!

Nutrition:

calories 300	fat 12g	fiber 8g	carbs 11g	protein 25g

68. Simple and Healthy Spinach Chips

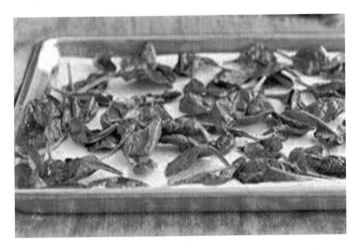

Preparation time: 10 min.	Cooking time: 10 min.	Servings: 3

Ingredients:
- 2 cups baby spinach
- A pinch of garlic powder
- ½ tablespoon extra-virgin olive oil
- Salt and black pepper

Directions:
1. Wash and pat dry baby spinach leaves; after, spreads them on a lined baking sheet.
2. In a bowl, mix oil with salt, pepper and garlic powder and whisk well.
3. Drizzle this over spinach, toss to coat, spread leaves again and bake in the oven at 325 degrees F for 10-12 minutes.
4. Leave spinach chips to cool down before serving.

Bon Appetite!

Nutrition:

calories 75	fat 4g	fiber 1.5g	carbs 2.4g	protein 2g

69. Broccoli "Cheese" Sticks

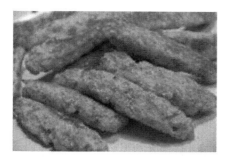

Preparation time: 20 min.	Cooking time: look the recipe	Servings: 22 sticks

Ingredients:
- 4 cups broccoli florets
- 1 cup almond flour
- ¼ cup coconut flour
- ¼ teaspoon onion powder
- ¼ teaspoon garlic powder
- ½ teaspoon salt
- 1 large egg
- ½ teaspoon apple cider vinegar (check the label for sugar additives)

Directions:
1. Preheat oven to 375 degrees. After, add the broccoli florets in a pot with boiling water. Boil for 8-10 minutes, until broccoli is soft, and drain the water.
2. Add the broccoli to a food processor and pulse until it is a paste-like. Transfer it into a bowl.
3. In another bowl, combine the almond flour, coconut flour, onion powder, garlic powder, and salt together. Add it to the broccoli, then add the egg and vinegar and mix well.
4. Pour the mixture on a parchment-lined baking sheet and place another piece of parchment paper over the top. Using a rolling pin, spread the down by pressing it out on the top piece of parchment paper until it's roughly ⅓ - ½ inch thick.
5. Remove the top piece of parent paper. Using a pizza cutter, score the dough to make sticks and after that put them into the oven for 30 min.
6. When a ready, leave them to cool, then break into sticks.
7. Place in the fridge. You can freeze any leftover sticks and thaw when needed.

Bon Appetite!

Nutrition:

calories 110	fat 3g	fiber 3g	carbs 11g	protein 5g

70. Special Zucchini Hummus

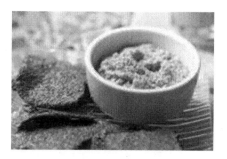

Preparation time: 10 min.	Cooking time: 20 min.	Servings: 6

Ingredients:
- 2 zucchinis, chopped
- 1 tablespoon coconut oil
- 4 garlic cloves, chopped
- ½ cup tahini
- 2 tablespoons lemon juice
- 4 ounces roasted peppers, chopped
- Salt and black pepper to the taste

Directions:
1. Spread zucchinis on a baking sheet, add salt, pepper, and the oil, toss to coat and bake in the oven at 400 degrees F for 20 minutes.
2. Take zucchinis out of the oven, leave aside to cool down for 10 minutes and transfer to your food processor.
3. Add more salt and pepper, tahini, garlic, lemon juice and roasted peppers and blend well.
4. Serve with veggies on the side after you've kept in the fridge for a few hours.

Bon Appetite!

Nutrition:

calories 140	fat 1g	fiber 2g	carbs 6g	protein 8g

Chapter 6: Dinner Recipes

71. Thai Coconut Chicken

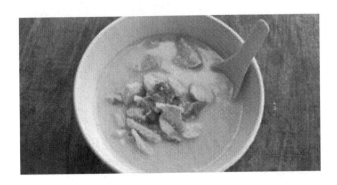

| Preparation time: 5 min. | Cooking time: 30 min. | Servings: 4 |

Ingredients:
- 1 pound chicken breasts (boneless, skinless)
- 2 garlic cloves, minced
- 1 cup onion, diced
- ½ cup sliced white mushrooms
- ½ cup carrots, sliced into coins
- 1 cup zucchini, sliced into half-moon shapes
- 1 can full-fat coconut milk
- 3 teaspoon green curry paste
- ½ teaspoon salt
- 1 tablespoon red chili pepper slices
- 1 tablespoon coconut oil

Directions:
1. Combine coconut milk with the green curry paste in a small bowl. Set aside.

2. Preheat a large, high-sided skillet with a lid, to medium-high and melt the coconut oil in the pan.
3. Meanwhile, cut the chicken breasts into 2-inch (5-cm) cubes. Season one side with salt.
4. Place the cubed chicken into the pan. Do not stir it. After 5 minutes, turn the cubes to a second side to sear for another 3 minutes.
5. Reduce the heat to medium, add the carrots, onion, and garlic. Cook and stir for about 4 minutes. Add the zucchini, mushrooms, chili pepper slices and salt. Keep stirring for another 5 minutes.
6. When the zucchini and mushrooms are brown, pour in the coconut milk mixture. Simmer for 10 minutes.
7. It is ready to serve!

Bon Appetite!

Nutrition:

calories 211	fat 6g	fiber 5g	carbs 12g	protein 35g

72. Delicious Zucchini Noodles with Turkey

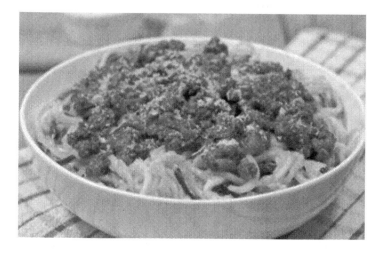

Preparation time: 10 min.	Cooking time: 20 min.	Servings: 4

Ingredients:

- 1 pound turkey meat, ground
- 1 tablespoon garlic, minced
- 3 tablespoons olive oil
- 28 ounces canned tomatoes, crushed
- 2 tablespoons tomato paste
- ½ cup yellow onion, chopped
- 3 zucchinis, cut with a spiralizer
- Salt and black pepper to the taste

Directions:

1. Heat up a pan with 2 tablespoons oil over medium high heat, add onion and garlic, stir and cook for 3 minutes.

2. Add turkey meat, salt, and pepper, stir and cook until the meat is done.

3. Add tomato paste and tomatoes and stir and cook for 10 minutes.

4. Heat up another pan with the rest of the oil over medium heat, add zucchini noodles, stir and cook for 2 minutes.

5. Divide noodles on plates, add turkey mixture on top.

Bon Appetite!

Nutrition:

calories 340	fat 12g	fiber 4g	carbs 26g	protein 30g

73. Savory Beef Chili

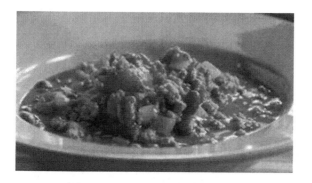

Preparation time: 10 min.	Cooking time: 5 hours	Servings: 6

Ingredients:
- 1 green bell pepper, chopped
- 1 pound beef, cubed
- 1 yellow onion, chopped
- 4 carrots, chopped
- 26 ounces canned tomatoes, chopped
- 1 teaspoon onion powder
- 1 tablespoon parsley, chopped
- 4 teaspoons chili powder
- 1 teaspoon garlic powder
- 1 teaspoon sweet paprika
- A pinch of cumin
- Salt and black pepper to the taste

Directions:
1. Heat up a pan over medium high heat, add beef, brown for a few minutes and transfer to your slow cooker.
2. Add bell pepper, carrots, onions and tomatoes and stir.
3. Also add salt, pepper, onion powder, parsley, chili powder, paprika, garlic powder, and cumin. Stir, cover and cook on high heat for 5 hours.
4. Divide into bowls and serve.

Nutrition:

calories 274	fat 6g	fiber 1g	carbs 32g	protein 24g

74. Chicken Meatballs with Herbs

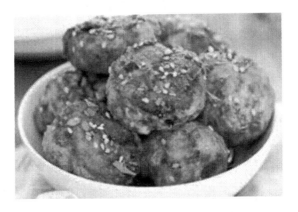

Preparation time: 10 min.	Cooking time: 25 min.	Servings: 6

Ingredients:
- 2 celery ribs, chopped
- 1 teaspoon ghee
- 1 and ½ tablespoons chicken meat, ground
- 3 garlic cloves, minced
- 1/3 cup almond flour
- 1 small yellow onion, chopped
- 2 tablespoons hot sauce
- ¼ cup chicken stock
- 1 cup green onions, chopped
- 1 cup parsley, chopped

- Salt and black pepper to the taste

For the sauce:
- ½ cup chicken stock
- ½ cup hot sauce
- 2 tablespoons coconut aminos
- 3 tablespoons ghee
- A pinch of black pepper
- 1 teaspoon garlic powder

Directions:

1. Heat up a pan with 1 teaspoon ghee, add garlic, onion, and celery, stir, cook for 5 minutes and take off heat.

2. In a bowl, mix chicken with the veggies, almond flour and 2 tablespoons hot sauce and stir well.

3. Heat up the same pan from the veggies over medium high heat, add ¼ cup chicken stock and heat up.

4. Shape meatballs from the chicken mix, drop them in hot stock, cook for 7 minutes, flip, cook for 7 minutes more and transfer them to a plate.

5. Heat up the same pan 3 tablespoons ghee over medium heat, add ½ cup stock, ½ cup hot sauce, coconut aminos, 1 teaspoon garlic powder, a pinch of black pepper and stir well. Simmer for 5 min.

6. Place back meatballs to pan and cook for 4 min. more. Divide between plates and serve with green onions and parsley on top.

Bon Appetite!

Nutrition:

calories 245	fat 4g	fiber 10g	carbs 9g	protein 8g

75. Grilled Salmon with Avocado Salsa

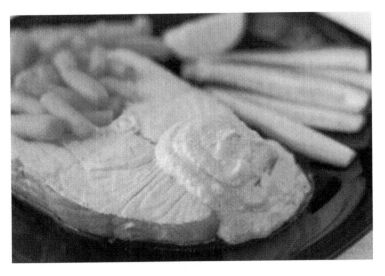

Preparation time: 10 min.	Cooking time: 25 min.	Servings: 4

Ingredients:
- 2 lbs. salmon, cut into 4 pieces
- 1 tablespoon olive oil
- 1 teaspoon salt
- 1 teaspoon ground cumin
- 1 teaspoon paprika powder
- 1 teaspoon onion powder
- 1/2 teaspoon ancho chili powder
- 1 teaspoon black pepper

For the Avocado salsa:
- 1 avocado, sliced
- 1/2 red onion, sliced
- 2 lemons (juice)
- 1 tablespoon cilantro, finely chopped
- Salt

Directions:

1. First, make the seasoning mix – combine the salt, chili powder, cumin, paprika, onion and black pepper. Then, rub the salmon fillets with olive oil and this seasoning mix. Put in the fridge for 30 minutes.
2. Preheat the grill.
3. Mix the avocado, onion, cilantro, lime juice, and salt in a bowl.
4. Grill the salmon until it's ready (about 5-7 minutes)
5. Top with avocado salsa and serve.

Bon Appetite!

Nutrition:

calories 140	fat 3g	fiber 4g	carbs 11g	protein 15g

76. Two Meat Salad with Mushrooms

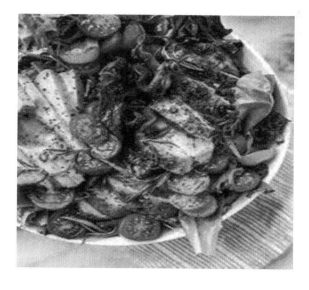

Preparation time: 10 min.	Cooking time: 10 min.	Servings: 4

Ingredients:

- 4 bacon slices, chopped
- 1 red bell pepper, chopped
- 2 sweet potatoes, baked and chopped
- 1 yellow onion, chopped
- 12 ounces cremini mushrooms, chopped
- 2 garlic cloves, minced
- ½ teaspoon thyme, dried
- 3 cups chicken, already cooked and shredded
- 2 cups spinach, chopped
- ½ cup olives
- Balsamic vinegar (check the label for sugar additives)
- Olive oil
- Salt and black pepper

Directions:
1. Heat up a pan, drizzle with a bit of olive oil, add bacon, brown for a few minutes and mix with onion, boiled potato pieces, garlic, bell pepper, mushrooms, thyme, and chicken.
2. Stir, cook for 10 minutes and season with salt and pepper to the taste.
3. Add spinach, stir, and take off heat.
4. Drizzle olive oil and vinegar over them and serve.

Bon Appetite!

Nutrition:

calories 230	fat 2g	fiber 8g	carbs 7g	protein 23g

77. Aromatic Beef Stew

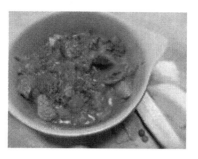

Preparation time: 20 min.	Cooking time: 45 min.	Servings: 4-6

Ingredients:
- 2 pounds beef stew
- 1 big yellow onion, roughly chopped
- 3 carrots, chopped
- 3 celery stalks, chopped
- 2 quarts beef or chicken broth
- 4 potatoes, cubed
- Extra virgin olive oil
- 2 garlic cloves
- ½ cup cremini mushrooms
- 1 32 ounces can of peeled tomatoes
- Herbs – dill, cilantro, basil (everything you like)

Directions:
1. Heat up a sauté' pan with olive oil, put garlic in, stir and fry for 1-2 minutes.
2. Add beef, brown from both sides. When it is ready, drain the liquid off and set aside.
3. Wipe pan clean quickly, add some more olive oil to the pan, and turn the heat on. Add onion, carrot, celery stalks, and sauté'. Add beef, stir it well and keep sautéing.
4. Take out a 16-quart stockpot. Add 2 quarts of broth. After, add the potatoes, mushrooms, and peeled tomatoes.

5. Simmer on the stove for 45-55 minutes.
6. Top with herbs and serve.

Bon Appetite!

Nutrition:

calories 320	fat 12.2 g	fiber 4.6 g	carbs 27 g	protein 26g

78. Turkey Burger on Eggplant Bun

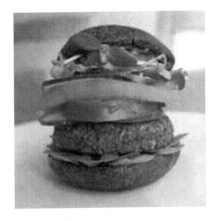

Preparation time: 10 min.	Cooking time: 15 min.	Servings: 4

Ingredients:
- 1 and ¼ pounds turkey, ground
- 1 sweet potato
- ½ cup spinach, frozen
- ½ teaspoon onion powder
- ½ teaspoon garlic powder
- Olive oil
- Salt and black pepper to the taste

For the eggplant buns:
- 1 large eggplant
- 1 tablespoon olive oil
- Salt and pepper

Directions:
1. Heat up sweet potatoes in the microwave for 4 minutes, peel and finely chop.
2. In a bowl, mix turkey meat with sweet potato, spinach, onion, and garlic powder. Add some salt and pepper, stir well and shape your burgers.
3. Heat up your grill over medium high heat, add turkey burgers, spray them with some olive oil and cook for 5 minutes on each side or so.
4. Preheat the oven to 425°F.
5. Line a baking sheet with foil. Cut one eggplant into 3/4-inch-thick rounds. Arrange in a single layer on the prepared pan. Drizzle 1 1/2 tablespoon of olive oil over the eggplant, then flip each slice and drizzle the remaining oil on the other side. Season with the salt and pepper. Roast the eggplant for 20 minutes, until it is browned on the outside and fork-tender. Leave to cool down.
6. Fill the space between two eggplants buns with the burger and serve.

Bon Appetite!

Nutrition:

calories 210	fat 12g	fiber 1g	carbs 0g	protein 24g

79. Delicate Steak and Peaches Dish

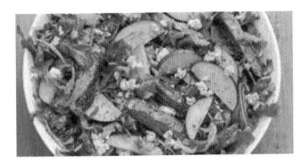

Preparation time: 10 min.	Cooking time: 20 min.	Servings: 2

Ingredients:
- 2 peaches, chopped and 2 slices reserved
- 3 handfuls kale, chopped
- 8 ounces filet mignon beef steak, sliced in half
- 1 tablespoon ghee
- A drizzle of olive oil
- A splash of balsamic vinegar (check the label for sugar additives)
- Salt and black pepper

Directions:
1. Heat up a pan with the ghee over medium high heat; add steaks and peach slices, fry well on both sides and transfer to a plate.
2. In a bowl, mix kale with chopped peaches (2 reserves slices), olive oil, vinegar, salt, and pepper. Stir well.
3. Thinly slice steak, add to salad and toss to coat.
4. Serve with grilled peach slices on top.

Bon Appetite!

Nutrition:

calories 260	fat 5g	fiber 4g	carbs 12g	protein 6g

80. Easy Seafood Paella

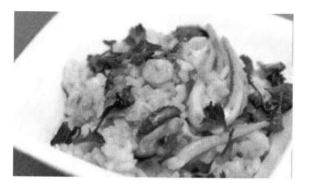

| Preparation time: 15 min. | Cooking time: 30 min. | Servings: 4 |

Ingredients:
- 1/2 lb. fresh shrimp, peeled and deveined
- 12-14 steamed mussels
- 1/2 lb. chorizo, sliced (check the label for sugar additives)
- 1 head cauliflower, grated
- A pinch saffron
- 1 yellow onion
- 1 red bell pepper
- 7 asparagus spears, chopped into bite sized pieces
- 3/4 cup water
- Olive oil
- Salt and pepper to the taste

Directions:
1. Grate the cauliflower and set aside
2. Chop onion, bell pepper, asparagus. Slice chorizo.
3. In a skillet with some olive oil, cook onion and chorizo until onion starts to turn translucent. Add chopped asparagus and bell pepper and cook until onion is thoroughly translucent and chorizo is cooked through. Set mixture aside.

4. In the same skillet, add cauliflower and saffron, salt, pepper, and 3/4 cup water. Cover and simmer for 5-7 minutes. Remove lid, stir, and cook for 5 minutes more. Add the sausage and vegetables to the cauliflower and stir to combine.

5. Meanwhile, steam mussels for 5 minutes. Discard any mussels that do not open. Cook your shrimp in another skillet with some olive oil – just for a few minutes, otherwise you will end up with rubbery shrimp.

6. On a platter, arrange mussels and shrimp atop cauliflower rice.

Bon Appetite!

Nutrition:

calories 343	fat 10g	fiber 2g	carbs 38g	protein 20.5g

81. Ruddy Pork Chops

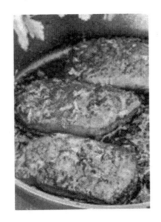

Preparation time: 10 min.	Cooking time: 15 min.	Servings: 5

Ingredients:

- 5 pork chops
- 1 tablespoon chili powder
- ½ teaspoon cumin
- ½ teaspoon chipotle chili pepper
- 1 teaspoon paprika
- 1 garlic clove, minced
- 1 cup coconut milk
- 1 teaspoon liquid smoke (make sure it does not consist any non-compliants)
- ¼ cup cilantro, chopped
- 1 lemon (juice)
- 2 tablespoons olive oil
- Salt and black pepper to the taste

Directions:

1. In a bowl, mix pork chops with salt, pepper, chili powder, paprika, cumin, chipotle chili pepper and garlic and rub well.

2. Heat up a pan, add pork chops, cook for 5 minutes on each side.

3. Meanwhile, in your food processor, mix coconut milk with chili pepper, liquid smoke, and cilantro. Blend well.

4. Pour this over pork chops in the pan, cook for a few minutes more and divide between plates. Drizzle lemon juice all over the chops and serve.

Bon Appetite!

Nutrition:

calories 200	fat 8g	fiber 1g	carbs 10g	protein 12g

82. Baked Buffalo Chicken Casserole

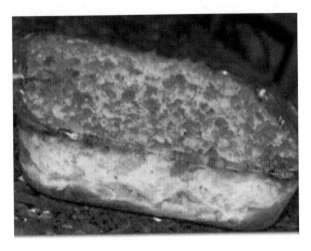

Preparation time: 25 min.	Cooking time: 1 hour	Servings: 4-6

Ingredients:
- 1 lb. chicken breast, cooked and shredded
- 3 3/4 cup cauliflower, riced
- 1 onion, diced
- 1/2 cup carrot, diced
- 1/2 cup celery, diced
- 1/2 garlic clove, minced
- 1 tablespoon ghee
- 1/2-3/4 cup buffalo sauce
- 1/2 cup egg whites
- 1 cup chives, chopped

Directions:
1. Preheat oven to 400 degrees.
2. Line a baking pan with parchment paper. Add onion, ghee, carrots, celery, and garlic to a skillet and sauté until onion is translucent and softened.

3. In a bowl, mix the cauliflower rice, shredded chicken, sautéed veggies, egg whites, and buffalo sauce.
4. Pour into lined baking pan and bake covered for 30 minutes.
5. After remove cover and bake an additional 20-25 minutes.
6. Top with chives.

Bon Appetite!

Nutrition:

calories 153	fat 13 g	fiber 4 g	carbs 13 g	protein 24 g

83. Stuffed Cabbage Patties with Pumpkin Sauce

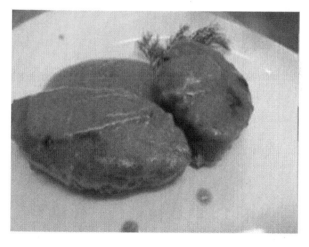

Preparation time: 30 min.	Cooking time: 45 min.	Servings: 6-8

Ingredients:
- 6-8 large cabbage leaves

- 1 pound ground beef
- 3 cups cauliflower, grated
- 1 tablespoon ghee
- 3/4 cup onion, diced
- 1 egg, whisked
- 1 teaspoon salt
- 1/2 teaspoon black pepper
- 1 teaspoon ground cinnamon
- 1/2 teaspoon garlic powder
- 1/2 teaspoon nutmeg
- 3/4 bottle pumpkin sauce (make sure it does not consist any non-compliants)

Directions:
1. Boil cabbage leaves for a few minutes and set aside to cool.
2. Preheat oven to 350 degrees F. Cook beef, onions, and ghee with all the seasonings in a medium skillet until no pink remains. After, drain any fat.
3. Add in cauliflower rice and egg.
4. Spread pumpkin sauce into the bottom of a lined pan. Remove any thick stem on cabbage leaves
5. Lay the cabbage leaf flat and add 1/3 cup filling to the center of the leaf. Roll cabbage leaf up like a burrito.
6. Pour remaining pumpkin sauce over the cabbage, cover with foil and bake 50 minutes.
7. Leave to cool down and serve.

Bon Appetite!

Nutrition:

calories 210	fat 5 g	fiber 2 g	carbs 30 g	protein 11 g

84. Classic Roast Chicken

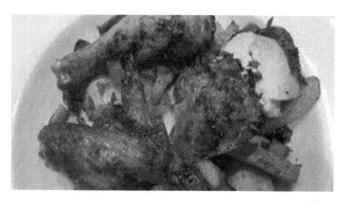

Preparation time: 10 min.	Cooking time: 1 hour and 10 min.	Servings: 4

Ingredients:
- 1 whole chicken, washed, pat dried and giblets removed
- 1 tablespoon salt
- ½ teaspoon black pepper
- 1 tablespoon ghee
- 1 shallot, chopped
- 2 teaspoons mustard (check the label for sugar additives)
- 1 cup chicken stock
- 2 teaspoons lemon juice
- 2 teaspoons tarragon, chopped
- Salt and black pepper

Directions:
1. Place chicken in a roasting tin, season with salt and pepper and rub well. Brush chicken with melted ghee, tie legs with kitchen twine, introduce in the oven at 425 degrees F for 30 minutes. After, flip it and roast for 30 minutes more.

2. Transfer chicken to a platter and leave aside for 20 minutes.

3. Meanwhile, let's make a sauce. Put 1 tablespoon cooking fat from the bird into a pan and heat up over medium heat. Add shallot, stir and cook for 5 minutes. After add stock and mustard, stir and bring to a boil. Finally, add tarragon, lemon juice, salt, and pepper, stir and cook for 5 minutes more.

4. Take sauce off heat and drizzle over the chicken before serving.

Bon Appetite!

Nutrition:

calories 300	fat 4 g	fiber 4 g	carbs 29 g	protein 27 g

85. Beef Steak Salad with Herbs

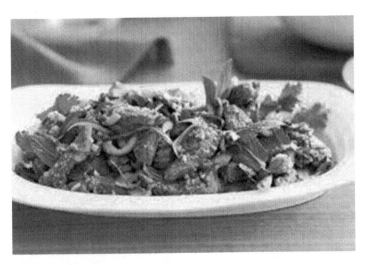

Preparation time: 10 min.	Cooking time: 20 min.	Servings: 4

Ingredients:

- 2 cucumbers, sliced
- ¾ pound sirloin beef steak
- 1 cup cilantro, chopped
- 1 cup dill, chopped
- 1 cup basil. chopped
- 1 shallot, chopped
- 1 teaspoon ghee
- 3 garlic cloves, minced
- 2 tablespoons coconut aminos
- 1 red chili pepper, chopped
- 2 teaspoons red pepper sauce
- 3 tablespoons lime juice
- Salt and black pepper

Directions:

1. Heat up a pan with the ghee over high heat, add beef steak, salt, and pepper, cook for 3-5 minutes on each side and transfer to a bowl.
2. In a bowl, mix garlic with chili pepper, aminos, and red pepper sauce. Stir well. After, heat up a pan, add dressing you've made and stir well. Then add lime juice, stir, take off heat and transfer to a bowl.
3. Slice beef steak and put in a bowl.
4. Add cilantro, cucumber, shallot, dill, and basil.
5. Add the dressing, toss to coat and serve.

Bon Appetite!

Nutrition:

calories 307	fat 23 g	fiber 12 g	carbs 4 g	protein 33 g

86. Slow Roast Beef

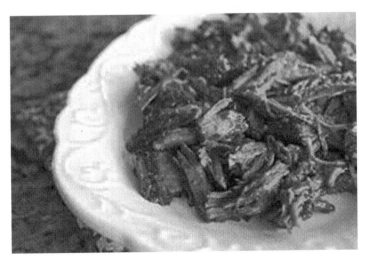

Preparation time: 10 min.	Cooking time: 8 hours	Servings: 6

Ingredients:
- 4 pound roast
- 6 garlic cloves, minced
- 1 yellow onion, chopped
- ½ cup balsamic vinegar (check the label for sugar additives)
- 1 cup chicken stock
- 2 tablespoons coconut aminos
- Salt and black pepper
- A pinch of red chili pepper flakes

Directions:
1. Put the roast in a Crockpot and add pepper, salt, garlic, onion, stock, vinegar, aminos, and chili flakes. Stir, cover and cook on Low for 8 hours.

2. After it's done, transfer roast to a cutting board and leave aside.

3. Transfer cooking juices to your blender and pulse well.
4. Slice roast and divide between plates.
5. Top with gravy and serve.

Bon Appetite!

Nutrition:

calories 255	fat 7g	fiber 1g	carbs 23g	protein 32g

87. Hot Pork with Beef Chili

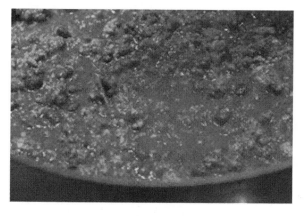

Preparation time: 10 min.	Cooking time: 2 hours	Servings: 8

Ingredients:
- 6 bacon slices
- 1 pound beef meat, ground
- 1 pound pork meat, ground
- 2 pounds sweet potatoes, chopped
- 1 yellow onion, chopped
- 1 tablespoon chili powder
- 1 teaspoon cumin

- ½ teaspoon garlic powder
- ½ teaspoon oregano, chopped
- ½ teaspoon cinnamon
- 1 bunch kale, chopped
- 1 cup water
- 2 avocados, pitted, peeled and chopped
- 2 limes, cut into wedges
- ½ cup cilantro, chopped
- Salt and black pepper + a pinch of cayenne pepper

Directions:

1. Heat up a pan over medium-high heat and brown bacon until it's crispy, transfer to paper towels, drain grease and chop.

2. Heat up the same pan with bacon fat, add sweet potatoes and onion, stir, cook for 15 minutes and transfer to a bowl.

3. Heat up the pan again, add beef and pork, stir and brown for a few minutes. Add salt, pepper, oregano, cinnamon, cumin, garlic powder, and cayenne and stir.

4. After, pour water, add potatoes and onion, stir and cook for 1 hour.

5. Add kale and bacon, stir and cook for 15 minutes more.

6. Divide into bowls and serve with avocado and cilantro on top and lime on the side.

Bon Appetite!

Nutrition:

calories 300	fat 7g	fiber 6g	carbs 32g	protein 18g

88. Spicy Shrimps with Cauliflower Puree

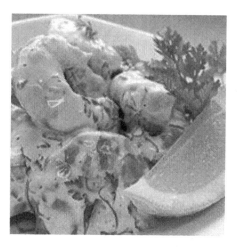

Preparation time: 10 min.	Cooking time: 2 hours	Servings: 8

Ingredients:
- 1 pound large shrimps, peeled and deveined
- 2-3 tablespoons Cajun seasoning (combine the salt, oregano, paprika, cayenne pepper, and black pepper in a plastic bag and shake to mix)
- 2 tablespoons ghee
- 1 12-ounce bag frozen cauliflower
- 1 garlic clove, chopped
- 2 tablespoons ghee
- Salt

Directions:
1. Bring to a boil water in a medium saucepan. Place cauliflower in a steamer basket and top with chopped garlic. Cover and steam until tender.

2. After, transfer cauliflower to the food processor and add ghee. Blitz until you get your desired consistency.

3. Make your shrimp. Pat dry and sprinkle with Cajun seasoning.

4. Heat 2 tablespoons ghee in a large skillet, add shrimp and cook 1-2 min. Flip the shrimp and cook until the bottom side is turning pink. When the shrimp are no longer translucent, remove from the skillet.

6. Transfer cauliflower into bowls and top with half the shrimp. Pour the ghee and spicy sauce from the skillet over serving bowls and serve.

Bon Appetite!

Nutrition:

| calories 340 | fat 14 g | fiber 5 g | carbs 16 g | protein 34 g |

89. Simple Chicken Salad with Egg

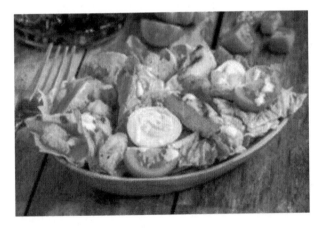

| Preparation time: 40 min. | Cooking time: 0 min. | Servings: 6-8 |

Ingredients:

- 1 chicken fillet (pre-cooked and chopped into small pieces)
- 12 eggs, hard boiled
- 1 celery stocks, minced
- ½ cup homemade mayonnaise
- 1 tablespoon yellow mustard (check the label for sugar additives)
- ½ cup chives
- Salt and pepper to the taste

Directions:

1. Chop boiled eggs into small pieces and place in the large bowl.

2. Add chopped chicken.

3. Add in mayonnaise, mustard, salt, pepper, celery, and chives. Stir gently and transfer to the fridge for a few hours.

Bon Appetite!

Nutrition:

calories 380	fat 28 g	fiber 0.5 g	carbs 2.8 g	protein 27 g

90. Tomato Quiche with Potato Crust

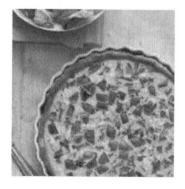

Preparation time: 10 min.	Cooking time: 1 hour	Servings: 4

Ingredients:
- 2 and ½ tablespoons ghee
- 2 cups sweet potatoes, grated
- 8 cherry tomatoes, cut in quarters
- 1 sweet onion, chopped
- 4 bacon slices, chopped
- 1 handful arugula leaves
- 6 eggs
- 3 garlic cloves, minced
- Salt and black pepper

Directions:
1. Spread sweet potatoes on the bottom of a pie pan, introduce in the oven at 450 degrees F and bake for 20 minutes.
2. Heat up a pan over medium high heat, add bacon, stir and cook until it browns. After, transfer to paper towels and drain excess grease.
3. Heat up again the pan, add onions, stir and cook for 5 minutes.
4. Add arugula and tomatoes, stir and cook for 4 minutes. Then, add garlic, stir, cook for 1 minute and take off heat.
5. In a bowl, mix eggs with salt, pepper, bacon and all the vegetables and stir.
6. Pour this over potato crust, introduce in the oven at 350 degrees F and bake for 30 minutes.
7. Serve hot.

Bon Appetite!

Nutrition:

calories 200	fat 5g	fiber 3g	carbs 12g	protein 9g

Chapter 6: Desserts Recipes

91. Baked Almond Butter Banana "Boats"

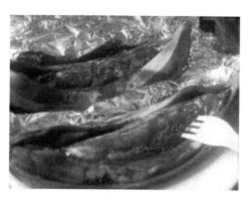

Preparation time: 3 min.	Cooking time: 15 min.	Servings: 1

Ingredients:
- 1 large banana
- ½ teaspoon cinnamon
- 1 tablespoon almond butter

Directions:
1. Preheat your oven to 375 degrees. Cut about ½ deep down the length of the banana.
2. Widen the cut with a spoon, making a place for the almond butter.
3. Fill in with the butter. Sprinkle with cinnamon.
4. Wrap completely in foil and bake for 15 minutes.
5. Allow it to cool for a few minutes, unwrap and serve.

Bon Appetite!

Nutrition:

calories 206	fat 9,4 g	fiber 5,3 g	carbs 31 g	protein4,7 g

92. Five-Minute Cranberry Nuts Bites

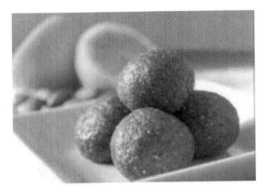

Preparation time: 5 min.	Cooking time: 5 min.	Servings: 16 bites

Ingredients:
- 1 cup almonds
- 1 cup cashews
- 1 cup dates
- 1 cup dried cranberries 130 g
- 1 teaspoon vanilla bean powder
- 1 lemon (zest + juice)
- 1/4 teaspoon salt

Directions:
1. In a food processor, put the cashew and almonds until coarse. Then add dates, cranberries, vanilla bean powder, lemon and salt and blitz until blended.

2. Roll into bite-sized balls. Place in an airtight container in the fridge for 30 minutes.

Bon Appetite!

Nutrition:

calories 125	fat 7 g	fiber 2 g	carbs 15 g	protein 3 g

93. Coconut Berry Mix Tarts

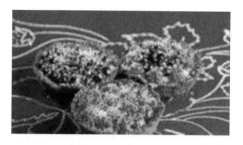

Preparation time: 5 min.	Cooking time: 5 min.	Servings: 16 bites

Ingredients:
- 14 medjool dates, pits removed
- ¼ cup almonds
- 1 can coconut milk
- ¼ cup raspberries
- ¼ cup strawberries, sliced

Directions:

1. In a food processor, put almonds and dates and process for about 1 minute until there are no big chunks.

2. Line two small springform pans with parchment paper. Divide the mixture between the two pans and with hands press it to form a crust.

3. In a bowl, put coconut milk and whip it for a minute with a hand mixer, then add the spoonful of the mixture that you've made and 5 raspberries. Beat until combined.

4. Put the coconut cream into the tart crusts and then top the tarts with raspberries and strawberries.

Bon Appetite!

Nutrition:

calories 110	fat 5 g	fiber 1 g	carbs 11 g	protein 1 g

94. Blueberry Banana Cream

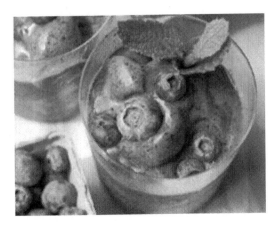

Preparation time: 5 min.	Cooking time: 5 min.	Servings: 4

Ingredients:
- 3 cups frozen bananas
- 1 cup frozen blackberries
- 1 tablespoon fresh mint

Directions:
1. Peel and chop bananas prior to freezing.
2. In a food processor, blend banana, blackberries, and mint until smooth and creamy. If necessary, allow bananas to thaw for a few minutes before blending. Serve immediately.

Bon Appetite!

Nutrition:

calories 90	fat 0 g	fiber 4 g	carbs 22 g	protein 1,5 g

95. Mango Chia Pudding

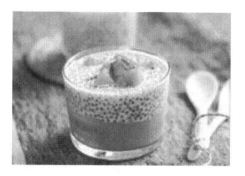

Preparation time: 10 min.	Cooking time: 10 min.	Servings: 4

Ingredients:
- 1 can of coconut milk
- ¼ cup chia seeds
- 2 mangos, peeled and mashed into a puree
- 2 limes

Directions:
1. Pour the coconut milk into a bowl and whisk thoroughly. Add the chia seeds and stir thoroughly to combine. Leave the chia pudding in the fridge for at least 4 hours but preferably overnight.
2. Divide the mango puree into four small bowls, reserving about 2 tablespoons as a topping.
3. Top all the bowls with chia pudding.
4. Grate lime zest on the top of the chia pudding.
5. Cut the lime into wedges. Squeeze them over the chia pudding. Serve with additional sliced lime wedges.

Bon Appetite!

Nutrition:

calories 86	fat 2 g	fiber 5 g	carbs 15 g	protein 1 g

96. Banana Almond Brownie

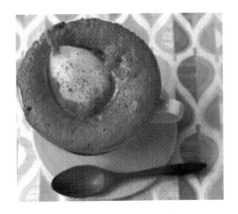

Preparation time: 1 min.	Cooking time: 10 min.	Servings: 1

Ingredients:
- 1 large ripe banana
- 1 tablespoon almond butter
- 1 tablespoon cocoa powder
- A pinch coconut flakes

Directions:
1. Mash your ripe banana, then add almond butter and cocoa powder and mix very well.
2. Grease a mug with some butter, transfer the banana mixture and top with coconut flakes.
3. Bake in an oven for 10-12 minutes at 350 degrees until cooked.

Bon Appetite!

Nutrition:

calories 135	fat 7 g	fiber 3 g	carbs 17 g	protein 1,8 g

97. Baked Cinnamon Apples with Sweet Potato

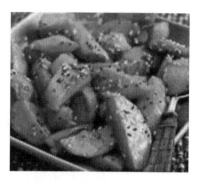

Preparation time: 1 min.	Cooking time: 10 min.	Servings: 1

Ingredients:
- 2 apples, sliced
- 2 sweet potatoes, peeled and sliced into rounds
- 2 tablespoon ghee
- 2 tablespoon water
- 2 teaspoon cinnamon
- Salt

Directions:
1. Preheat oven to 375°F. In a casserole dish, put apples, potatoes, ghee, cinnamon, and water. Mix until apples, and sweet potatoes are evenly coated.
2. Cover with foil and bake in the oven for 30 minutes.
3. Toss sweet potatoes and apples through baking time.
4. Remove foil, stir and bake for 15-20 minutes more tossing again halfway through baking time.
5. Remove from oven, sprinkle with a little salt and serve.

Bon Appetite!

Nutrition:

calories 140	fat 5 g	fiber 3,8 g	carbs 22 g	protein 1 g

98. Fruit Popsicles

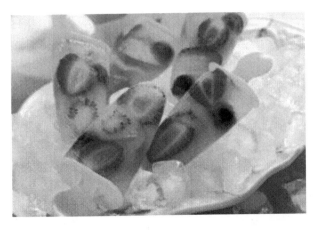

Preparation time: 1 min.	Cooking time: 10 min.	Servings: 1-3

Ingredients:
- Coconut water (check the label for sugar additives)
- Fruits of your choice (banana, blueberries, melon, kiwi, grapes, pear), chopped

Directions:
1. You need popsicle molds/form. Place all fruits into the molds, leaving room for the sticks of a popsicle.
2. Pour in coconut water, but do not fill to top since the liquid will expand during the freezing.
3. Put them in the freezer until set.

Bon Appetite!

Nutrition:

calories 90	fat 0 g	fiber 1 g	carbs 23 g	protein 0 g

99. Pumpkin Walnut Custard

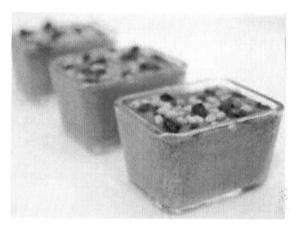

Preparation time: 5 min.	Cooking time: 50 min.	Servings: 4

Ingredients:
- 2 lb. 5 oz. pumpkin, baked and pureed
- 4 eggs
- 1 teaspoon cinnamon
- 1 teaspoon ginger
- 1/2 teaspoon nutmeg
- 1 can coconut milk
- 2 teaspoon vanilla bean powder
- 1 teaspoon pumpkin spice
- ¼ cup walnuts, chopped
- Coconut oil
- 1 tablespoon ghee butter
- Salt

Directions:
1. Preheat oven to 350°F. Combine pumpkin, coconut milk, eggs, cinnamon, ginger, pumpkin spice, and nutmeg in a bowl. Add a pinch of salt.

2. Beat on high until all ingredients are well combined.

3. Grease 4 custard dishes with coconut oil. Pour in pumpkin mixture and bake in the oven for 30 minutes.

4. In a small bowl, combine walnuts, ghee butter, and vanilla bean powder. Microwave until melted and stir to combine.

5. Add topping to the center of custard and bake for another 20 minutes. Leave custard to rest in oven for a little bit to prevent it from cooling too quickly.

6. Put in the fridge for 4-5 hours to cool prior to serving.

Bon Appetite!

Nutrition:

calories 108	fat 7 g	fiber 3,3 g	carbs 6,3 g	protein5,9 g

100. Sautéed Apples with Coconut Butter

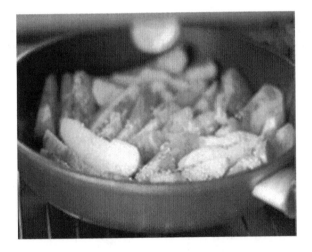

Preparation time: 2 min.	Cooking time: 10 min.	Servings: 2-3

Ingredients:

- 1 large apple, peeled and sliced
- 1 large pear, peeled and sliced
- 1-2 tablespoon coconut oil
- 2 teaspoon ground cinnamon
- ¼ teaspoon sea salt
- 3 tablespoon coconut butter, melted

Directions:

1. Heat a medium nonstick skillet and add 1 tablespoon of the coconut oil

2. Once heated, add the apples and cook/stir one minute, then add the pears and combine.

3. Sprinkle the salt over the top and stir, continue to cook until softened, about 3 minutes, adding any extra coconut oil and making heat lower if you need to.

4. Lower the heat and sprinkle the cinnamon over apples and pears, stir. If the mixture is very sticky, you can add a drop of water to thin it out. Once the fruit is coated with cinnamon, soft and lightly browned, remove from heat.

5. Microwave coconut butter in a glass for 5 sec until drippy but not too hot. Drizzle over apples and pears to serve.

Bon Appetite!

Nutrition:

calories 105	fat 5 g	fiber 2,5 g	carbs 8 g	protein 2 g

Conclusion

As you can now see, the Whole 30-day diet system is not so hard to follow. It is very simple and diverse at the same time, and there are so many amazing dishes you can cook, making yourself as well as your family happy.

I hope that these special 30 days will make you a healthier and happier person. But definitely, it will change the way you live and of course, the way you cook!

Thank you for reading!

Enjoy your food!

Enjoy your life!

And the most important – love yourself – beautiful and unique, no matter your size, no matter your weight

Made in the USA
Middletown, DE
18 April 2018